the
ULTIMATE
TEA DIET

the
ULTIMATE

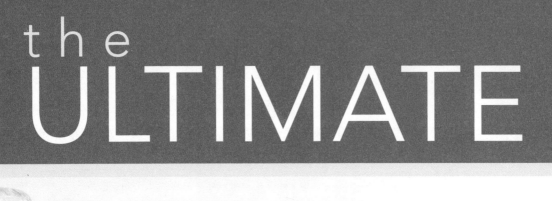

Your Guide to Good Health
One Cup of Tea at a Time

TEA DIET

How TEA Can

 * *Boost Your Metabolism,*

 * *Shrink Your Appetite,* and

 * *Kick-Start Remarkable Weight Loss*

Mark "Dr. Tea" Ukra

with Sharyn Kolberg

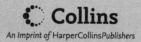

Collins
An Imprint of HarperCollinsPublishers

PAULINE HAASS PUBLIC LIBRARY

This book will educate the reader about the health benefits of drinking tea. It is based on the personal experiences, research, and observations of the author, who is not a medical or naturopathic doctor. This book is intended to be informational and by no means should be considered a substitute for advice from a medical or naturopathic professional, who should be consulted by the reader in matters relating to his or her health and before beginning any diet or health program. The author and publisher expressly disclaim responsibility for any adverse effects arising from the use or application of the information contained in this book.

THE ULTIMATE TEA DIET. Copyright © 2008 by Mark Ukra. All rights reserved. Printed in the United States of America. No part of this book may be used or reproduced in any manner whatsoever without written permission except in the case of brief quotations embodied in critical articles and reviews. For information, address HarperCollins Publishers, 10 East 53rd Street, New York, NY 10022.

HarperCollins books may be purchased for educational, business, or sales promotional use. For information, please write: Special Markets Department, HarperCollins Publishers, 10 East 53rd Street, New York, NY 10022.

FIRST EDITION

Designed by Jaime Putorti

Library of Congress Cataloging-in-Publication Data has been filed for.

ISBN: 978-0-06-144175-2

07 08 09 10 11   WB/RRD   10 9 8 7 6 5 4 3 2 1

DEDICATION

To my entire family, both living and in our hearts. To Gram and Grampa, Mom and Dad, Sis, Curly Lulu, and Mo. To every person seeking to make a change in their lives. To my daughter Lucky and my most loving and devoted wife and best friend Julie, whose guidance provided the catalyst for this guide.

CONTENTS

the
ULTIMATE
TEA DIET

INTRODUCTION

I never set out to write a diet book.

My wife and I own a shop in Los Angeles called dr. tea's. Every day, people come in just to enjoy a cup or two of tea, maybe read a book, do some work in a peaceful atmosphere, or chat with friends. Sometimes they see me in my bright orange lab coat or apron and we start to talk. And they tell me their troubles. Now, I'm not a doctor, or a shrink, or even a bartender, but people tend to speak to me about what's going on in their lives. Many have a vague notion that tea is good for you, but don't know why or how. In only two years of owning dr. tea's, I've had thousands of conversations about tea.

The one subject that has kept coming up over and over again is: "What tea can I drink to help me lose weight?" And I tell them about tea and the fact that it has three amazing ingredients that work together on the body's chemistry to increase metabolism, decrease appetite, and help stabilize blood sugar. I'd show them the *Camellia sinensis* plant, the plant from which all true tea comes, and tell them that any tea—White, Green, Oolong, or Black—that comes from this plant will help them lose weight.

I explained to them what has worked for me, and that it could work for them, too. People began to follow my plan, and they lost weight. And they told their friends, who came into dr. tea's wanting to know my "secret." I gave them the same information, they would tell their friends—and you know how that goes. I soon realized that the best thing for me to do was to write down my "tea" story and spread the word.

Thus *The Ultimate Tea Diet* was born.

A tea diet? Really? I don't blame you for being skeptical. I would be, too—if I were to say that all you had to do was drink tea and the pounds would come flying off. No such luck. Tea is miraculous in many ways, but it is not a miracle drug. If you want to lose weight, you have to be able to say: "I can lose weight, eat a balanced diet, and exercise a moderate amount." But you don't have to go to extremes, and you don't have to be perfect every single meal for the rest of your life. You do have to eat proteins, fats, and carbohydrates (yes, carbohydrates). The Ultimate Tea Diet will show you how to easily judge proportions and portions of these nutrients without a scale or a calorie counter. You'll get a 14-day meal plan you can follow as is, or use as a guideline to make your own healthy breakfasts, lunches, snacks, dinners, and even desserts. And, oh yes—the recipes! You may be surprised to learn that you can not only drink tea, you can cook with it, too.

I am proof positive that the Ultimate Tea Diet works. But I am not the only proof. I now have hundreds of "test-TEA-monials" from people just like you who've lost both weight and inches by following the simple diet and drinking tea all day. In fact, you can get started on The Ultimate Tea Diet right now, before you read another word, just by finding a tea you love and drinking it all day—in the morning, at noontime, in the evening, before meals, with meals, after meals. Drink it hot, drink it cold, drink it however you like. Just start drinking tea and you will begin to see and feel a difference.

This book is devoted to everyone who feels hopeless, disheartened, and just plain tired of the way they look and the way they feel. There's no mumbo-jumbo here, it's all backed up by science. All you have to do to begin is find a tea you love and start drinking.

When I began drinking tea, I began to feel healthier and happier about myself! I began to take control of my life—you will start to take control of yours. The simple act of making an educated, well-thought out choice about what you ingest all day, each and every day, will be your ticket to making all of the changes you've wanted to make in your life.

You will probably start on this diet just to lose weight. You *will* lose weight and you *will* lose inches. But you will gain so much more. You will see differences in your skin and your hair. You will want to be more active and begin working out, and you will feel sharper and a lot more energetic. And you will get back the confidence you once had and have somehow lost along the way. And I can confidently say that to you, not only from my own experience, but from all the feedback I get from people who have gone on the Ultimate Tea Diet and have come back or emailed me at drtea@ultimateteadiet.com to tell me how much their lives have changed, one cup of tea at a time.

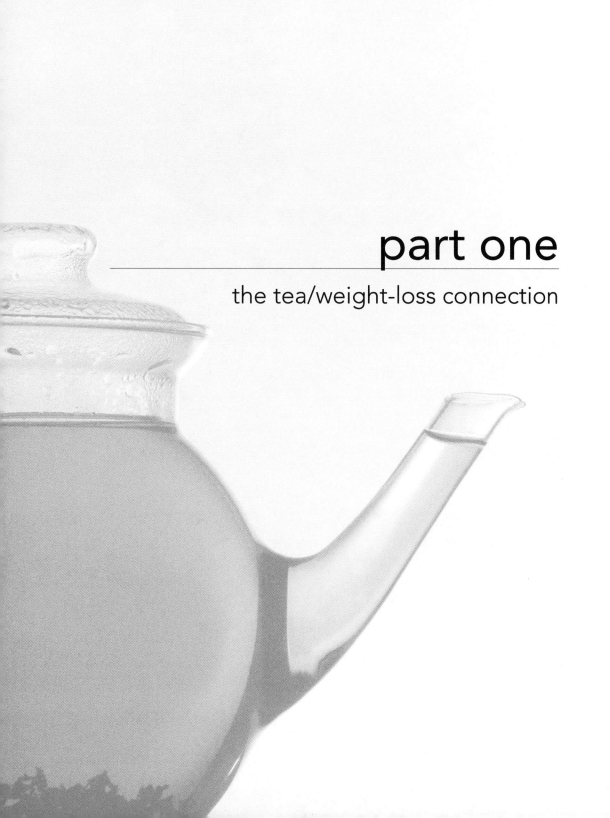

part one

the tea/weight-loss connection

1

What's Tea Got
to Do with It?

Dear Dr. Tea,

I have been heavy my entire life. I have a very supportive family and friendly coworkers, but when you don't like the way you look, nothing anyone says or does to make you feel better works. I was negative about myself and everyone around me.

Here's where you come in. Driving home from work I passed dr. tea's daily and always wondered what it was like. I stopped my car a couple of times, but the patio was full of "beautiful people" and I felt terribly inadequate, so I would slink away. One day on the drive home I was listening to a call-in show on the radio, and found myself listening to a woman with the same complaints and woes as I had—and she sounded truly pathetic.

I pulled over and cried for half an hour. Then I turned my car around and headed straight back to your store, walked past the people on the patio and found an empty seat at your tea bar. I started to ask you questions about the health benefits of your teas. You stopped me dead in my tracks when you started to talk about the amazing weight-loss benefits associated with tea. Then you began to tell me about your Lifestyle Diet, and I started to take notes.

I did just what you said. I drank my tea all day, ate what I knew was right for me to eat, meditated at least one minute a day, and started to do something in the form of exercise. I had not moved around much for years. I began by walking around the house and Dr. Tea, I have now made it around the block.

I am happy to tell you, I have lost 17 pounds in the last month. I feel healthier and happier than I have ever before. Thinking positively has changed everything about me. I owe you so much Dr. Tea. You treated me like I was somebody and now I am. May all of life's blessings visit you often.

Edith P., Los Angeles, CA

Edith P. is, like millions of Americans, concerned about her health, unhappy with her appearance, and insecure about her ability to change her life. When she came to me for advice, I told her to do the very thing that had worked for me: start slowly, stop the insanity of endless diet plans that do not work, and start your journey towards good health, one cup of tea at a time.

That's right, tea.

I am not a physician, a dietician, a nutritionist or a psychiatrist. I am just a regular guy, like you, who figured things out for himself fifteen years ago. I am an expert on and aficionado of tea. My family has been in the tea business for over 200 years. I have studied everything there is to study on the subject, and I have traveled the world to learn tea firsthand. I have tasted and tested nearly every kind of tea there is, from tea bags to prized tea cakes that have been aged for decades, from teas mixed with yak butter to teas served in the finest china.

And here's what I know: *It's tea's time!* According to the Tea Association of America, the tea industry topped $6.2 billion in 2005 (and is expected to exceed $10 billion by 2010) with Americans drinking 2.2 billion gallons of tea each year. Americans are wising up to the fact that they don't need a "grande" beverage from the local coffee establishment to get the extra boost they need to make it through their day. The health benefits of tea can provide the stimulation and kick without all the side effects of a highly caffeinated beverage. It's simply a cup of good health a day.

Do you know which beverage is the most consumed in the world? No, it's not coffee, or beer, or wine. It's water. And what comes next on the list? Still not coffee. Nor wine nor beer. It's tea. In the most populated countries in the world, the drink they consume most often after water is tea.

It's time for tea to be recognized in this country, not only for the health benefits most of the world have known about for centuries, but for its incredible ability to help stop one of the world's biggest health crises to date: obesity. Americans, and American children and teenagers, are getting larger and larger every year and are paying the consequences in diabetes, heart disease, and stroke.

Millions of Americans go on and off diets every day. If you're reading this book, you are probably one of those millions, and you are probably tired of your own yo-yo dieting experiences. We try to eat right, to make healthy choices, and to get off our addictions to sugar and caffeine, but it's just too hard.

So we turn to drugs; we buy supplements made from obscure plants found only in African deserts; we cut out entire food groups; and we get totally confused by what the latest diet guru is telling us to eat (which is just the opposite of what the previous guru espoused). What we don't know is that we don't need drugs, supplements, or slide rules to help us figure out how to shed the pounds. What we do need to know is very simple: *Drinking tea will help us lose weight.* Yes, tea. Inexpensive. Good tasting. And available to everyone everywhere. Tea, with *natural* ingredients that will not only help us lose weight, but will reduce our cravings for sweets, suppress our appetite, increase our insulin's effectiveness, lower our cholesterol, and stimulate thermogenesis, which helps the body burn fat for energy. All this from a cup of tea!

This is not theory, guessing, or wishful thinking. This is hard science, proven in study after study conducted over the past ten years by some of the most respected scientists around the world who have all come to the same conclusion: tea helps you lose weight.

Simple, and true.

How Does It Work?

The Ultimate Tea Diet is the first book to reveal tea's incredible weight-loss potential. The secret is the synergy of tea's three main ingredients: caffeine, L-theanine, and epigallocatechin-3-gallate (EGCG), which will all be explained fully in later chapters. But here's a quick rundown of the ingredients, starting with caffeine. Because caffeine is a stimulant, it will help you lose weight. Unfortunately, however, caffeine has unhealthy side effects. Recent studies have shown that caffeine raises both blood sugar and insulin levels.

Doesn't tea have caffeine?

Yes, it does, but it has far less than you'll find in a cup of coffee. And here's the "magic" of tea: It also has L-theanine, an amino acid that works to counter caffeine's harmful effects. L-theanine also influences the neurotransmitters in the brain that affect your dopamine and serotonin levels which send the brain signals of satiety. The more tea you drink, the stronger the message to your brain that says "I'm not hungry." Therefore, tea not only helps you lose weight, it helps you to reduce your appetite and stay on a diet as well.

The third secret ingredient of tea is EGCG, the miracle antioxidant that stimulates your body's metabolism; you're actually burning fats as you sit there drinking your tea. EGCG also lowers the levels of triglycerides in the blood and inhibits the accumulation of fatty acids in the fat cells, thus making it a significant antiobesity agent.

Can you eat whatever you want and still lose weight simply by adding tea to your diet? Probably not. But if you start by drinking tea, it will begin its work on your alpha brain waves, your neurotransmitters, and your metabolism to increase your energy and decrease your appetite. When you add in the Ultimate Tea Diet weight-loss food plan and a moderate amount of exercise, the pounds and inches will come off quickly and safely.

Okay, so right about now you're thinking, "Here we go again. Another diet book promising me this and that—only this one's about tea." Right?

Wrong!

The Ultimate Tea Diet is not just another diet book. No way! I'm as tired as you are of all of the diet books that make weight-loss claims; they may help you lose weight for a few weeks or months—and then you're right back to your current weight, or even worse, you're heavier than you were before, leaving you depressed and dejected because you could not stay on that diet.

Those diets work initially because of what you have to give up: sweets and snacks and sometimes whole categories of foods (missing those carbs, anyone?). On The Ultimate Tea Diet, you do have to cut back on sweets and snacks, but you also learn to eat healthy, balanced meals that include all food groups. But what makes this diet so unique is not what you have to give up, but what you add: the tea.

And that's not all. *The Ultimate Tea Diet* is a simple guide to making changes in your life that will allow you to lose weight. This is why it works, and why it will work for you as it has for me, and countless dr. tea's clients over the years.

> *A by-product of this lifestyle is losing weight and keeping it off.*
> *A by-product of this lifestyle is gaining control of your life.*
> *A by-product of this lifestyle is getting back the confidence that you lost oh-so-many diets ago.*
> *A by-product of this lifestyle is feeling energized all day.*
> *A by-product of this lifestyle is feeling healthier and happier.*

Success Stories

At the same time I started to write this book, I began to invite a group of people to go on The Ultimate Tea Diet journey with me. Eighteen intrepid TEAmmates followed the program for eight weeks, kept journals, answered weekly questionnaires, and lost a combined total of 197 pounds. It was a diverse group, ranging in age from early 20s to mid-50s, with a variety of weight-loss goals. It was more successful than we ever imagined it would be. We even had three members of the same family (two brothers and a sister) who together lost more than 60 pounds in just eight weeks! You'll meet some of these people throughout this book, and hear what they had to say. For instance, when asked after just the first week what was the most noticeable difference The Ultimate Tea Diet made, Christine A. answered:

My appetite! Wow . . . the first day drinking tea all day I wasn't even hungry for dinner. That NEVER happens to me! Tea really does suppress your appetite. I was afraid tea wouldn't work for me, but I was wrong. It does. I have added tea into my life and I love it.

There are several factors that make followers of the Ultimate Tea Diet so successful.

1. *Its basic tenet is easy to remember: find the teas you love and drink them all day.* One of the best things about the Ultimate Tea Diet is that tea comes in a huge variety of flavors and forms. In the next chapter, you'll learn to identify the types of teas that have the most weight-loss benefits—but within those categories you have literally hundreds of choices. There are sweet teas, pungent teas, salty teas, light teas, and heavy teas. There are fruity teas and spicy teas. There are teas in bags and teas in tins. There are teas that are relatively expensive, and teas that are extremely economical. If there's one thing I can guarantee, it's that with all these choices, you will be able to find many teas that you will not only like, but that you will look forward to drinking every day.

2. *The suggested food plan is easy to follow.* It's a healthy, balanced diet that includes proteins, carbohydrates, and fats, and even several tasty snacks and desserts. But the most exciting aspect of the plan is that everything in it is infused with tea! There are tea-based foods for breakfast, lunch, and dinner, sweet treats and midday snacks, all deliciously

made with tea so that you are getting the health and weight-loss benefits with every single bite you take. And they are scrumptious, to boot! And here's the beauty part: everyone knows that a lean breast of chicken is a nonfattening, healthy diet choice. But as anyone who's ever been on a diet will tell you, after a week of chicken breasts, you'd give up your firstborn for some smokey barbeque. Luckily, the Ultimate Tea Diet not only gives you a huge range of foods besides chicken—you can change the flavor of your food simply by changing the kind of tea seasoning you use. Want a smokey barbeque taste? Try using Lapsong Souchong. Like a tangy citrus kick? Rub on some Earl Grey (which is blended with oil of bergamot, a small acidic orange). The Ultimate Tea Diet includes dozens of recipes along with tips and techniques for choosing the tea that will give you the taste you want.

But the true beauty of the Ultimate Tea Diet is in the simple fact that tea can be added to any other diet or meal plan you are on and produce positive weight-loss results. So if you're on Weight Watchers, you can enhance your results by drinking tea all day and adding tea to Weight Watchers' recipes. If you're on the You on a Diet plan, or The Zone, or South Beach, or the Miami Mediterranean Diet, or Volumetrics, you can do the same. Not only will you lose weight if you follow The Ultimate Tea Diet, but simply by drinking tea all day, you can unlock the potential for any other diet plan to work as well.

3. *Dr. Tea's Weight-Loss Philosophy: If you want to make changes in your life, you have to change your thoughts and your habits.* There are several commonsense steps you can take to make that happen:

✴ *Say you can and you will! Say you can't and you won't.* Do not let saying "I can't" continue to be your excuse for not changing your life and losing weight. Say you can change your life, and you will! Say you can lose weight, and you will! If you want to change what you eat, you have to change how you think about your food. Focus your energy on drinking tea, eating right, and following the food plan, and you will lose weight.

✳ Drink tea all day so that your body is constantly metabolizing. Scientists agree that an average adult should consume between 2 and 2.5 liters of water per day (that's about eight to ten 8-ounce glasses). This intake needs to be increased during periods of hot weather, and during and after periods of physical activity. Your daily requirement doesn't have to be pure water, however. Tea counts just as well! I recommend at least eight 8-ounce cups a day. But most people on the Ultimate Tea Diet fill their 16- or 24-ounce water bottles, sip from them all day, and refill when necessary. As you read through the book, you'll find many ingenious methods of carrying and drinking tea morning, noon, and night.

✳ Plan your meals for the day. Everything we do starts with our thoughts. Start the day by thinking about the day's menu, and focus your energy on carrying out that plan.

✳ Identify the foods that trigger your bingeing. Everyone has foods that turn on the urge to overeat. For some people it's bread, for others it's ice cream, cookies, cake, or candy bars. Even though drinking tea will help curb those cravings, you have to know which particular foods will have you fighting against the tea's effects, and eliminate those foods from your pantry and your diet.

✳ Eat only when you're hungry and stop eating when you're full. We all eat for a variety of reasons. Learn to identify your eating habits (do you eat when you're anxious, happy, stressed, overtired?). Let your body tell you when you need to refuel for sustenance and energy, not for comfort or for relief of emotional pain.

✳ Replace any bad eating habits with a cup of tea. If you have to have something sweet before bedtime, try a caramel- or chocolate-flavored tea, or a tea infused with hints of apple, blueberry, or pumpkin pie (yes, Virginia, they do exist). If what you're about to eat is not on your plan for the day, find a suitable tea to replace it—and the pounds will begin to disappear.

If you want to get started on the diet right away, go directly to chapter 8. But please, come back and read chapters 2 through 4 so that you understand what a miracle tea is and why it will work for you. And be sure to read chapters 5, 6, and 7 so that you understand that you *can* lose weight, whether you've been successful at it before or not, by changing your thoughts and by finding the teas that are going to satisfy your cravings and make it easy for you to stay on the Ultimate Tea Diet.

It's my goal to make this journey as easy as possible for you. As with everything in life, the more you put into it, the more you get out of it. Don't expect yourself to be perfect, because none of us is perfect. You will have slip-ups, setbacks, and lapses in judgment just like I have. These are temporary. Relax and know that tea is forgiving, and all you have to do is go right back to the Ultimate Tea Diet because, as you will find out by reading the rest of this book, the key components of tea will actually help you stay on the diet. So if you are ready to make a change in your life, then go make yourself a cup of tea—or better yet, brew yourself a whole pot—and let's get started on the journey to a slimmer, healthier you, one cup of tea at a time. It's as easy as one—two—TEA.

> *It is very strange, this domination of our intellect by our digestive organs. We cannot work, we cannot think, unless our stomach wills so. It dictates to us our emotions, our passions. After eggs and bacon it says, "Work!" After beefsteak and porter, it says, "Sleep!" After a cup of tea . . . it says to the brain, "Now rise, and show your strength. Be eloquent, and deep, and tender; see, with a clear eye, into Nature, and into life: spread your white wings of quivering thought, and soar, a god-like spirit, over the whirling world beneath you, up through long lanes of flaming stars to the gates of eternity!"*
>
> JEROME K. JEROME (1859–1927):
>
> *Three Men in a Boat*

TEAmmate Profile

Name: **Ron H.**

Age: **37**

Total Weight Loss: **11**

Total Inches Lost: **9.75**

Favorite Tea: **Lemon Ginger**

I started getting heavy when I was in grade school. My parents kept pushing me to lose weight. The first diet I was on was similar to Weight Watchers. I had to go to meetings with my mom. I was the only kid there. We'd sit every day and count calories. I hated it. I went off that and gained weight again.

In college, I gained the usual freshman 15. Then I gained another freshman 15 and another freshman 15. My sophomore year I got really into running. I wasn't really on a diet, but that helped me lose weight. Then I came out to California. I had asthma, and coming out here set it off, so I stopped running. Of course, I got fat again.

I tried a couple of different diets here and there. I did the no-fat thing. I tried some kind of fat-burning soup diet. That was disgusting. I would lose a little and then go off it and go crazy and gain everything back.

When I about 34, I hit 300 pounds. I went on the Atkins diet and lost 125 pounds in nine months. I felt great and I was running six miles a day. I had to go buy new pants every couple of weeks. However, as soon as I let myself have some carbs again, I went right to the donut store. I snapped back up to 240. Then I got engaged and I had to look good for the pictures, so I lost 20 pounds doing South Beach. Then I got married, the pictures were taken, and I went back up to 260.

Last year, my first daughter was born. I started to have low back problems and knee problems and my asthma was acting up. I wanted to be there to see her grow up, and I wanted to be able to participate in whatever she wants to do. I had a newborn, and I wasn't sleeping, and my job was very stressful. Also, I had really bad digestive issues last year and I had to go see a gastroenterologist. He told me I had to clean up my diet, and cut back on the seven or eight cups of coffee I had been drinking every day.

Then I heard about Dr. Tea and the Ultimate Tea Diet. Now my life is very different. When I get up I walk my dogs with my daughter. When I get home from the walk, I have breakfast and make a big cup of green matcha tea. At around 11:00 a.m. I have some iced tea I made the night before. Then I have a glass of tea with lunch. Then a couple of hours after lunch, I have a snack and some more tea. After I eat dinner, I drink a couple of mugs of Lemon Ginger tea. It feels like when I wake up in the morning, my system is refreshed and ready to go.

Sometimes it's nice in the middle of the day to just take some time to have a cup of tea. And I like having the ritual of making tea. It takes up the space that food usually occupies in my head.

The biggest difference for me is that I have been able to cut out in-between-meal "grazing." It had always seemed to me that I would wake up in the morning and just start eating. I was always hungry. The Ultimate Tea Diet has focused me on having three distinct meals, and knowing that I can have a snack in the afternoon if I feel I need one. I'm also much more conscious now while I'm eating of how I'm feeling in terms of being full. That's something I'm more aware of when drinking the tea. I don't start off as ravenous, so I don't feel like I have to eat as much. Every time I eat, I try to have a protein, a carbohydrate, and a little fat, and not to have all of just one.

But one of the most freeing things Dr. Tea said was to let yourself have a bad day. And if you do, don't jump off the track. Think of this as a life change, not a fad diet where you're going to lose all this weight and something magical is going to happen. I've had bad days. Even just bad meals. But then later that day I can make a good choice and have another cup of tea.

Steeped in Knowledge:

A Short Primer on Tea

Not too long ago in America, a cup of tea was a cup of tea was a cup of tea. Now you can go into almost any supermarket and find dozens of brands and flavors from which to choose. This is good news and bad news. It's good because people are drinking more tea than ever, and that's what we want to happen. The bad news is that you may be confused—if not intimidated—by all the tea options and don't know how to make the right choice.

This chapter will help you out of your confusion.

Here's the first and perhaps the most important thing you need to know: Not everything you think of as tea is really tea. All true tea comes from one plant, *Camellia sinensis*. That's right! All tea comes from one plant. There is not a white tea plant, a green tea plant, an oolong tea plant, or a black tea plant. There is only one tea plant. Now you know more about tea than 95 percent of the rest of America does. So when you read about a medical study where green tea is proven to aid in weight loss, or if you read that white tea is good for reducing cholesterol, you now know that all tea comes from the *Camellia sinensis* plant, so it does not matter which type you drink.

I am often asked which kind of tea is the healthiest. My answer is always the same: "The kind you like to drink." There are some minor differences in the four kinds of tea: White teas and green teas have slightly higher levels of polyphenols (antioxidants found in plants); oolong and black tea have recently been shown to be more effective in preventing certain diseases, such as heart disease and high blood pressure. However, the general consensus is that the kind of tea you drink is not as important as the fact that you drink it.

All four types of tea have the *same* health benefits. All four types of tea will aid in your weight loss; all four types of tea will help reduce cholesterol. And all four types of tea have many more proven health benefits, which you'll read about in the next two chapters.

If the beverage you're drinking does not come from *Camellia sinensis*, it is not tea. "Tisane" (tee-SAHN) is the term used within the industry for anything that resembles tea but does not come from the tea plant. *When we talk about tea throughout the rest of this book, unless we specifically say otherwise, we are talking about the four main categories of tea that come from this plant: white, green, oolong, and black.*

This is important to remember because if you want to lose weight on the Ultimate Tea Diet, you must drink true tea. Only tea that comes from the *Camellia sinensis* plant contains the properties that will help you lose weight. Of course, if you want to drink tisanes in addition to true tea, go right ahead. Although they don't contain weight-loss aids, most have other positive health benefits. And many are extremely helpful for reducing cravings for sweet snacks, especially in the evening hours.

The Four Teas of *Camellia Sinensis*

If all true tea comes from the same plant, how are the different types created? What distinguishes one type of tea from another is the way the leaves and leaf buds are processed after harvesting; these processes vary somewhat from country to country, but the basic concepts are the same around the world. Because all tea comes from the *Camellia sinensis* plant, the differences are created by the length of time the tea leaves are allowed to "ferment," or oxidize.

White Tea

White tea, which has always been revered as the "Tea of Royals," is the most delicate and least processed tea in the world. White tea, named for the *hao*, or the white hair on the bud or baby leaf, is known for its mild flavor and natural sweetness. It is made from young leaves that have undergone no oxidation. The production of authentic white tea is restricted to a limited geographical area in southeastern China's Fujian province. In fact, it wasn't until the 1990s that white tea was introduced to the Western world. It possesses the least caffeine of all the tea types, and is prized for its cooling and refreshing character while delivering many antioxidant and heart-strengthening elements, and is becoming more and more popular as a result of the newfound health benefits.

White tea was being produced as far back as the Tang Dynasty (618–907 AD). At that time, the nature of the beverage and the style of tea preparation were quite different from the way we experience tea today. Tea leaves were processed into cakes and prepared by boiling pieces of the compressed tea in earthenware kettles. This special white tea of Tang was picked in early spring when the new growths of tea bushes that resemble silver needles were abundant.

The processing sequence for white tea is:

1. Leaves and buds are harvested.
2. Leaves and buds are cleaned.
3. Leaves and buds are dried.

Green Tea

During the Song Dynasty (960–1279 AD), production and preparation of tea changed throughout China. Even then, people were looking for convenience; a new form of tea emerged as a result of people wanting more and more tea without having to take the time to brew the leaves. The tea leaves were picked and quickly steamed to preserve their color and fresh character. After steaming, the leaves were dried. The finished tea was then ground into fine powders that were whisked in wide bowls. The resulting beverage resembled what we know of today as instant tea—you mixed the tea powder with hot water and voilà! Your tea was ready in an instant.

This tea was highly regarded for its deep emerald or iridescent white appearance and its rejuvenating and healthy energy. This style of tea preparation, using powdered tea and ceramic ware, became known as the Song tea ceremony. Although it later became extinct in China, this Song style of tea evolved into what is now the Japanese tea ceremony that endures still today.

Today, there are between 12,500 and 20,000 green teas produced in China alone (although they are named and renamed so many times—for no apparent reason—that no one knows exactly how many there are). It is similar to wine in that respect. There are thousands of vineyards that produce wines; not all of them make it to market, or are meant to do so. It's the same with tea in China. There are thousands of individual tea plantations and each produces its own variety of tea. Some are meant only for an individual farmer's consumption; others may be distributed in a local area; and still others are grown for the commercial market and shipped worldwide.

As with white tea, the bud and leaves for green tea are picked, cleaned, and dried. The tea leaves then undergo a minimal amount of oxidation. Green tea has very low levels of caffeine, and derives its distinctive, healthy good flavor from the area in which it is grown and the techniques used to produce the tea. The processing sequence for green tea is:

1. Leaves and buds are harvested.
2. Leaves and buds are cleaned.
3. Leaves and buds are dried.
4. In Japan, the leaves are steamed, which stops any fermentation.
5. In China, the leaves are placed in very hot woks to stop any fermentation.
6. The tea is then rolled, cut, ground, or shaped into a form uniquely associated with the plantation on which it is grown.

Dragon's Well is the most famous of Chinese green teas; it grows on the peaks of the Tieh Mu (t'yeh MOO) mountain range. Chinese mythology tells us that the dragon is the king of the waters. History tells us that in 250 AD, there was a drought at the Dragon's Well monastery. A monk prayed to the dragon, pleading for rain. His prayers were immediately answered, and the tea produced there received its name.

Oolong Tea

Oolong tea, referred to as the Champagne of teas, is a semioxidized whole-leaf tea, which retains all of the nutrients and natural healing factors contained in unfermented green tea, but without the raw, grassy taste. It falls somewhere between green and black tea, with complex flavor and aroma. The leaves go through a very brief fermentation process, which eliminates harsh irritants from the raw tea and creates the subtle fragrances and flavors that distinguish this tea from all other varieties.

Oolong legend tells us Wu Liang (who lived during the Ming Dynasty in China, around 1400 AD), a tea farmer, went out one day to pick tea, as he did every day in the tea-picking season. He had collected quite a bit when his eye was caught by a deer drinking by the river. He stopped his tea-picking activities and killed the poor animal (sorry to have to report this). He took the slain deer home, as it would provide him with a week's worth of meals. He forgot all about his tea. When he went back to collect his load, he found that the tea had started to blacken. We know today, it had begun to oxidize.

Wu Liang thought that it might have gone bad, but decided to proceed with his traditional preparations. He dried the tea by pan-firing, as was done with the green teas of the day. When he made a cup of this tea, he was surprised to find that it tasted different than his usual green tea, and discovered that he loved the flavor. He taught his neighbors and friends how to make the new tea, and it came to be named after him. Language being what it is, the name eventually evolved from Wu Liang to Oolong.

The processing sequence for oolong tea is:

1. Leaves and buds are harvested.
2. Leaves and buds are cleaned.
3. Leaves and buds are placed in bamboo containers and air is blown through them. This process is referred to as "withering the leaves."
4. The withered leaves are rolled, which releases the oils within the leaf. These oils mix with the oxygen in the air and the leaves begin to ferment or oxidize.
5. When the rolled leaves reach a dark blue-green color, they are placed into a hot wok to stop the fermentation process and add flavor.

Black Tea

Of the four tea types, black tea is allowed to oxidize the longest and is known for its beautiful red color and light sweet taste. (The Chinese call it red tea because the actual tea liquid is red; westerners call it black tea because the tea leaves used to brew it are usually black.) This process produces a hearty, deep, rich flavor. Black tea contains the most caffeine, but still has only about half the amount of a regular cup of coffee. About 75 percent of the tea produced worldwide is black tea; it is the type of tea consumed by 87 percent of American tea drinkers.

The processing sequence for black tea is:

1. Leaves and buds are harvested.
2. Leaves and buds are cleaned.
3. Leaves and buds are withered.
4. The withered leaves are cut and fermented.
5. When the cut leaves turn from blue-green to dark red or black, they are placed into the hot wok to stop the fermentation process and add flavor.

TEASER

Would You Pay $300 for a Pot of Tea?

The rarest and most expensive type of tea in the world is the mysterious Pu-Erh (poo-AIR) tea from the Pu-Erh region of China. Pu-Erh is an aged black tea prized for its medicinal properties and earthy flavor. Until 1995, it was illegal to import Pu-Erh into the United States, and its production process is still a closely guarded state secret in China. It is very strong; it has an incredibly deep and rich flavor, but it is not bitter. Black Pu-Erh tea has been fermented in a similar fashion to wine and cheese. In fact, black Pu-Erh is fermented, and then fermented again after the first fermentation process is stopped. This is what differentiates Pu-Erh from other black teas. Following the double oxidation process, the tea is pressed into a round or brick-shaped teacake. It is then left to mature for as much as fifty years (although there is much disagreement on the optimal number of years for the best flavor).

There are actually two types of Pu-Erh, black and green. Black Pu-Erh is the fermented tea, while green Pu-Erh is not fermented. In Tibet, Pu-Erh is sometimes boiled with yak butter, sugar, and salt to make yak butter tea. Pu-Erh tea can be found only in a few select tea shops in this country (including dr. tea's) and can cost as much as $1,000 an ounce, $300 for a pot, or $50 for a cup to go.

When a Tea Is Not a Tea

As I said earlier, true tea is that which comes from the *Camellia sinensis* plant. If it does not come from the plant I endearingly call "Cami," it isn't technically tea. It's like Champagne in that respect—in order to be called "Champagne," wine has to come from the Champagne area of France. If it comes from any-where else, it is technically referred to as "sparkling wine." Similarly, if a bever-age does not come from the *Camellia sinensis* plant, it cannot be called a "tea"—even though most of the world refers to any hot beverage that looks like, smells like, or tastes like tea—as tea.

There are a huge number of tisanes, or herbal drinks, that are commonly called tea. You see them every time you go into the supermarket, especially the ever-popular chamomile, peppermint, and lemon verbena. These herbal "teas" are, according to the Tea Association of America, ". . . an infusion of leaves, roots, bark, seeds or flowers of other plants [not *Camellia sinensis*]. They lack many of the unique characteristics of tea and are not linked with the research on the potential health benefits of traditional teas." These herbal drinks do not contain caffeine; they are generally made by pouring boiling water over the plant parts and letting them steep for a few minutes.

The Fuss About Rooibos

There is one tisane that has recently been "discovered" by tea lovers and is cur-rently garnering a lot of attention. A naturally decaffeinated beverage with high levels of antioxidants, it is known as Rooibos (ROY-bus) and it has been growing in South Africa in the Cederberg Mountains, just north of Cape-town, for centuries.

Rooibos does not come from Cami. The Rooibos plant is part of the le-gume family and is often described as being sweet with a slight nutty aftertaste. Since Rooibos contains less than half the tannin found in regular tea (tannins are a natural substance found in many plants, including grapes and tea leaves, that produce an astringent, mouth-puckering sensation) it is naturally sweet, and most people drink it without sugar. When brewed, Rooibos has a reddish brown color, perhaps explaining why it is sometimes referred to as "red tea."

There are two types of Rooibos, red and green. Green Rooibos (unmatu-rated) is harvested when the plant is still green. Red Rooibos is harvested when the Rooibos is turning from green to red. Both red and green Rooibos are cut out in the fields, similar in fashion to wheat, and taken to a factory.

When Rooibos is cultivated commercially, the needlelike leaves and stems are usually harvested in the summer, which corresponds to the months of January through March in South Africa.

The mild flavor of Rooibos, and the fact that it is naturally decaffeinated, has made it a popular component of herbal drinks that are blended with other ingredients, such as chocolate, caramel, ginger, and dried fruits.

TEASER

The Flavors of Tea

In chapter 7, you'll discover a number of ways to determine the kind(s) of tea that suit you best. In the meantime, my advice is to try as many varieties as possible. Remember that many teas are blended during processing to give them additional flavor. Green tea, for instance, may be blended with jasmine. Black tea may be sprayed with bergamot orange oil to make Earl Grey. At dr. tea's, we make both "regular" and decaffeinated versions of many teas so that orange, blueberry, or pineapple flavors (to name a few) can be consumed by people who want true tea (or who are on the Ultimate Tea Diet), and we mix many of the same flavors with Rooibos for people who are concerned about caffeine in general or who want a decaffeinated tea to drink at night.

Tea Comes in Many Forms

You will learn many things about tea as you read this book. One of the things you will learn is that there are several ways to buy tea. You can buy tea from a tea shop (there are shops all over the country these days); you can purchase tea over the Internet; and you can buy tea in grocery stores, convenience stores, and even pharmacies. That's not to mention every place you can get tea already brewed for you. Every dining establishment, from a five-star restaurant to a roadside diner and even the ubiquitous coffee shop, serves tea, both hot and cold.

When you are buying tea to brew at home, you can get it in two forms: loose leaf tea or tea bags. You are probably most familiar with tea bags. This is known as commercial grade tea, and it is made of *dust* and *fannings,* the by-products of the tea-making process. Dust is the tiniest particles of tea, and fannings are broken tea leaves one grade larger than dust. Here's the first thing you need to know about tea bags: You get the same health and weight-loss benefits from tea whether you brew it from dried loose tea leaves or from a paper tea bag, as long as it is white, green, oolong, or black tea. The second thing you need to know is that a paper tea bag is meant to be used only once (you will understand why that is important as you read on in this chapter). The flavor you get from a tea bag may not be as rich as the flavor from loose leaf teas, but the only way you will know which you like best is to do a taste test.

Loose leaf tea is just what it sounds like: tea that comes not in a bag, but as full or cut tea leaves. These are leaves and buds that are harvested and processed as explained above, and usually sold by weight. Because you are getting more surface area from loose tea than you get from dust and fannings, you usually get a richer flavor.

TEASER

The Who, What, Where, How, and When of Tea

It makes no difference *who* manufactures the tea; *what* type of tea you use (white, green, oolong, or black); *where* it comes from (tea bag or loose leaf); or *how* you serve it (hot or cold). But it does matter *when* you use the tea, as you never want to use stale tea. If your teas have been in the cupboard for a few years it's time to get some new tea. Most teas, if stored in a cardboard or paper container, will be good for a year. If stored in a metal container, tea will stay fresh for two years.

Brewing the Perfect Pot of Tea

There is much more to learn about tea. But I imagine that if you're reading this book, you're most concerned about losing weight. So here's what I suggest you do: If you haven't already done so, brew yourself a cup or a pot of tea. Don't be concerned if you don't have high-quality loose leaf tea sitting in your cupboard. You probably have a tea bag somewhere back there. If that's the case, start by drinking that. Then go out and purchase some loose leaf tea (if you can't find a tea shop near you, there are plenty of Web sites that offer tea online), and make up a pot.

Some people are intimidated by the thought of brewing loose leaf tea, only because they've never done it before. It's easy; in fact, it's easier than making a pot of coffee. Always remember that the perfect pot of tea is personal to the drinker; you have the finest nose and palate, and the way you brew your pot of tea is the best for you. Do not get caught up with all of the hoopla about steeping time and water temperature—just get to it.

Here's the short explanation of how to brew tea: Heat some water, pour a little of the hot water into a teapot, swish it around, and throw it away. Then put enough tea leaves in the pot to entirely coat the bottom of the vessel with a thin layer of tea. Not an inch of tea, but a thin layer of tea (about $1/16$ inch). Let steep for two minutes or so, strain, and enjoy.

TEASER

Making Oolong Tea

Oolong tea requires a slightly different preparation than the other three teas. White tea is harvested as a whole leaf, so it is easy to see how much is coating the bottom of your vessel. Green and black tea leaves are cut during processing, but you can still easily see how much is at the bottom. Oolong tea, however, is a whole leaf that has been rolled; you therefore coat only half of the vessel with tea because when you add the hot water, the tea in the pot will double in size. Coating the entire bottom with oolong will place too much tea into your vessel. The same goes for any tea (oolong or not) that is rolled, such as Jasmine Pearl or Gunpowder.

Your vessel is defined as whatever touches your tea leaves during the preparation. So if you are using a teapot, then the pot is your vessel. If you are using a strainer, then the strainer is your vessel and not the cup into which you put the strainer.

For those of you who want a little more detailed instruction, just follow the suggested steps below:

1. Start with fresh cold water in a saucepan or tea kettle. Do not use hot tap water to begin the boiling process as this will affect the taste of the water. Try to find the best bottled spring water, or use filtered tap water.

2. Preheat your teapot: Pour some of your hot water from the tea kettle or from the hot-water spout in your water cooler into the teapot, swish it around, and then discard the water. You do this so that the hot (non-boiling) water will not cool down too quickly as it hits the tea, and to allow your loose leaf tea to open up and relax before pouring in the hot water. You see, tea is just like us. When we get into bed at night and the sheets are cold we curl up a bit and wait until we adjust to the coolness of the sheets and then stretch out. If tea leaves are placed into a cold vessel they do the same thing; they curl up and wait to relax until they adjust to the temperature. When we immediately add very hot water to the vessel, the tea leaves go into shock. As you can imagine, this will affect the smell and taste of the tea leaves (not to mention your enjoyment).

3. Then add your loose tea to the teapot or strainer as explained earlier. Do not use too much tea. You can always add more tea to your next steep.

4. Tea balls: Most tea experts frown on the use of balls because they do not allow the tea leaves room to expand, which gives tea its best flavor. This is the same criticism the commercial grade of tea bags receives. When you feel you need something else to make your tea, buy it. But there's no need for you to run right out and buy a bunch of tea accessories; I'd much rather you get started making tea with whatever you have on hand. If you do use the ball, please fill it only halfway with your tea to allow for complete saturation and expansion of the tea leaves.

TEASER

Choose a Little Teapot . . .

Choosing the proper cookware can influence the way your meal turns out. Some people like to cook in a wok because once it's seasoned, the wonderful oils and flavors of everything you've previously cooked in it will be included in each new culinary creation.

The same goes for tea ware—the teapot you use can impact the flavor of your tea. Some people like to use metal teapots specifically for the "wok effect." If you prepare tea in a metal pot, the pot will absorb the flavor of the tea. So if you brew a pot of black tea in metal and then brew white tea in the same pot, the white tea will take on some of the black tea notes.

Personally, I like to use a glass teapot. Glass does not absorb the flavor of the tea as it is being brewed; neither do china or ceramic pots. So you can brew any kind of tea and the next pot won't be infused with the flavor of the one before. But this book is all about you. Use the teapot you love; your tea will be perfect for you and that's all that matters.

5. Pour your hot water over the tea and cover (leave uncovered if you want it to cool faster). Some people believe that the water has to be boil*ing* (not boil*ed*) when it hits the tea leaves and that if it's merely hot then the tea will be insipid. Wrong! Do not use boiling water; it destroys the flavor of the tea and lessens the flavors of your additional steeps.

6. Steep your tea according to your taste. An easy way to remember the steep time is to start with steeping all teas for 2 to 3 minutes. You will always have a great tea and you can think of the other matters in your life while the tea is steeping, or maybe just close your eyes and concentrate on your breathing for 2 to 3 minutes. If you feel the taste of the tea is too weak, add more tea to your next steep. Do not steep the tea longer to make it stronger. If you do, you pull out all the wonderful flavor and leave less for the next steeps you make. If the taste is too strong, reduce the amount of tea in your next steep.

7. While your tea is steeping, rinse your teacup or mug with hot water, the same way you rinsed the teapot.

8. If you like to drink your tea with milk in it, pour the milk into the cup before you pour in the brewed tea. This keeps the milk from curdling or coagulating. Now, an important note for you milk lovers: there is currently some controversy over whether or not it is good to put milk in your tea. A recent German study seemed to prove that putting milk in tea reduced and in some cases eliminated the antioxidants we need in our tea to assist with weight loss and good health. However, in an article titled "Brewing Up the Latest Tea Research," published by the United States Agricultural Research Service, Dr. Jeffrey Blumberg, associate director of the USDA Human Nutrition Research Center on Aging stated, "There has been only one study showing that adding milk decreased the bioavailablity of catechins in tea. Those results were not replicated in any of several subsequent studies." A Scottish study published in May 2007 measured participants' blood levels for antioxidants after drinking tea without milk, and then did the same thing

again after having them drink tea with milk. This study found that adding milk made no difference to the beneficial properties. So here's my advice: drink your tea the way you like it! And, if you are worried about adding milk, you might want to switch to rice or almond milk so you can be completely sure you're preserving the antioxidants in your tea and still enjoy the milklike quality. Or you can give your favorite tea its own milklike flavoring by adding Tahitian vanilla beans or extract to your cup or pot (this is a great tip for people who can't have dairy).

9. Before pouring the tea, shake the teapot a little and then let the tea leaves settle again. Now pour the liquid into your favorite cup or mug.

10. Taste the tea, and then add sweetener or lemon if necessary. You put the sweetener or lemon in last for the same reason you taste a meal before you add salt (you don't put salt at the bottom of the plate and then put your meat over it). Some teas are sweeter than others and you may not need to add anything at all. And every cup or pot of tea you brew will be different from the last—you may have added a pinch more or less tea, or let it steep for a few more seconds. These factors will change the taste. If you do use sweetener and don't want to use sugar, agave (a honey-like substance from the cactus plant), or honey, I recommend and urge that you stay away from the chemicals in those blue, pink, and yellow packets and try stevia, a noncaloric natural sugar substitute that you can find at any health food store, instead.

TEASER

Concerned About Caffeine? Resteep Your Tea

Although you'll learn a lot more about caffeine as you read through this book, here's something most Americans don't realize: You can steep your tea leaves over and over again. Whether you make a pot of loose tea or use a noncommercial tea bag (commercial tea bags are produced to be used once and thrown away), you can re-use it several times (loose tea more than bagged tea). *And the caffeine virtually disappears after the first steep.* So if you don't want the caffeine, follow the steps above to brew your tea, but don't drink the first pot. Pour that liquid down the drain and most of the caffeine will go with it! Or refrigerate the liquid, and use it to make caffeinated iced tea at a later time; use it for cooking (see the Tea Rice recipe on page 193); or you can even use it to water your plants.

If you're using a noncommercial tea bag (some high-quality loose teas come in special silk or nylon bags), you can reuse it twice or three times. But when you use quality loose leaf tea not in bags, you can resteep the leaves a minimum of four times, up to ten or twelve times. You can even resteep the tea several times, refrigerate the pot overnight, and use the leaves again the next day. Be sure to discard these leaves after the second day; otherwise they may grow harmful bacteria.

If you have a garden or indoor plants, just throw your used leaves on the ground or into the indoor pot to use as mulch. Your plants will love you for it!

12. If you are using a tea bag instead of loose tea, use one bag per cup. Just like loose tea, however, you always put the tea bag in first, then add the water. Many restaurants serve it incorrectly—they give you a cup of hot water with a tea bag on the side and you are expected to dip the bag into the cup. You will find that when you drop the bag into the water, it will float on top. The water doesn't saturate the tea, so you must use your spoon to push the tea bag down into the water. If you are serving it at home, pour the milk into the cup, if you like it that way, then place the tea bag in the cup, then pour in the water. Lastly, add sweetener or lemon if necessary.

Shopping for Tea

When I look at loose tea I am looking for freshness and the ability to resteep my leaves many times. These are my criteria:

1. Smell: Does it smell fresh? Or is the "nose" gone? If there is not much smell you can assume that the taste is also depleted.

2. Look: If it is possible to see the tea leaves, ask yourself, "Do they look fresh? Do they look dried out or stale?" If there are flavors added, how are they added? For instance, if it is a Green Pineapple Tea, are there bits of pineapple in it, or have they added pineapple flavoring? Dried fruit means more care went into the mixing and may also indicate that the tea is of a finer quality. But I have many clients who prefer the taste of the flavors to the real fruit, so it is really a matter of taste. If you are in a tea shop, always ask for a sample before you buy any quantity of the tea. If you are ordering online, purchase a small quantity for your first order, especially if you have never used that supplier before.

3. Buying tea in bags: There are several different kinds of tea bags available. Some tea makers put loose leaf teas in silk or nylon bags. We make some of these at dr. tea's. These are meant to be used one to a cup, and may be used for one or two steeps. Most commercial bags are made of paper, and meant to be used once. Read the labels on boxes of tea bags so you know what you are getting. I recently saw two boxes in the grocery store with very similar names. One was called Tiger Spice, and one was called Bengal Blend. Both had pictures of tigers on the box. However, one was true tea and one was not. The ingredient label on Tiger Spice read, "Black tea, cinnamon, ginger, roasted chicory" and several other flavors. That told me that black tea was the main ingredient. The ingredients listed on the second box, Bengal Blend, were "cinnamon, roasted chicory root, roasted carob, ginger" and several other flavors. After reading that label, I knew it was an herbal blend (tisane) and not a tea.

4. This is a time to experiment also and see which ones are best for you. Find a local teahouse and get familiar with their wares. Or go online and start a chat with the tea purveyor. Remember if they do not have time to answer your questions about their products, then they probably do not take the time to create a great tea.

Hot Out? Have a Nice Iced Tea

There is nothing more refreshing on a hot day than an ice-cold glass of iced tea. The good news is that it's really easy to make. If you just want to make one glass for yourself, brew yourself a pot following the directions above, let it cool a bit, and then pour it over ice. What could be easier?

If you want to make a big old jug-full for the family, or for the week, you'll need two large pots—like the one in which you usually make spaghetti. In the first pot, boil up your water; remove it from the burner. Coat the bottom of the second pot with your loose tea (or throw in several tea bags, depending on how strong you want your tea). Pour your hot water into your second pot (the one with the tea in it) and let it steep for 2 to 3 minutes.

Place a fine strainer on top of the first large pot (now empty) and pour the tea liquid back into it. Let the tea cool, and then pour into your favorite jug or jar. There you have your iced tea. Pour it over ice, or put into the fridge to have later.

But don't discard those leaves—you can reuse them to make another batch of iced tea, or several pots of hot tea. Remember, any kind of tea can be made into iced tea. And if you want a special treat that tastes like a smoothie or a Slurpee, make yourself what we at dr. tea's call a Frostea. Just pour your brewed tea over ice in a blender, add a little agave or honey, and blend away (turn to chapter 11 for some flavorful Frostea recipes). I've found that children love this cold treat—and it's much better for them than soda pop or sweetened fruit juice.

Remember that you may want to make your tea a little stronger than usual, as the ice cubes will dilute the tea as they melt. On the other hand, if you've made a batch of tea and it is a little weaker than you would like, you can always make your ice cubes out of tea (page 254) and plop them in your glass!

The best quality tea must have creases like the leathern boot of Tartar horsemen, curl like the dewlap of a mighty bullock, unfold like a mist rising out of a ravine, gleam like a lake touched by a zephyr, and be wet and soft like a fine earth newly swept by rain.

LU YU (733–804 AD),

The Classic of Tea

TEAmmate Profile

Name: Amber Z.

Age: 28

Total Weight Loss: 12

Total Inches Lost: 12

Favorite Tea: Pineapple Coconut White Tea

This has been a rough couple of years for me. And I've tried every kind of diet there is, and my weight has yo-yo'd tremendously. Because of that, I started having major gallbladder problems. Then I went on an all-vegan diet. I lost weight and my gallbladder healed, but then I thought, okay, now I'm better—so I just started eating everything again.

I gained a bit of weight, but I was doing pretty well. Until about four and a half years ago, when I got a job at Starbucks. I had a lot of stress in my life. I was taking care of my grandmother who was ill with cancer. I was working from four in the morning until one in the afternoon. I never had breakfast and I barely had lunch. At the end of the day, I might make myself a healthy dinner, but maybe not. All day long I would be hopped up on caffeine just to keep myself awake and keep myself full. I figured at least I wasn't smoking, so I was fine.

I actually became very irritable and nervous. My fiancé kept asking, "What's happening to you?" I gained 45 pounds in the first year of working there. I maintained it for four years. I went from 140 to 198. I felt miserable. I started to change my eating habits. I started eating healthier foods. I was having oatmeal in the morning, I was having a healthy lunch. And I still wasn't losing weight. I'd maybe lose 4 pounds. I was so sluggish. I never felt good. I was always run down.

When I was drinking coffee all day long, I felt terrible and I went into depression physically and mentally. Right before I started the tea diet, I quit my job. Now that I've lost the weight, I feel great. I don't think I would have normally been able to handle planning a wedding and looking for a new job. But something about drinking the tea would keep me on an even keel during the day. Now, when I'm upset, instead of going to the cupboard and grabbing something to eat, I grab a cup of tea. And my fiancé is now saying, "My girlfriend's back!"

For a while, I really had no self-confidence. I have to say, this diet totally changed my life. For me, it's not even a diet. It's a way of thinking. As Dr. Tea always tells us: If you say you can, you will; if you say you can't, you won't. And I actually have that quote right next to my bed so when I get up it's the first thing I see.

I recently got a job working at a women's gym. Two months ago, I never would have believed I'd be working at a gym. I started as a receptionist but I just got a promotion about a week ago and I am now head of sales coordinating and marketing. And yes, I associate it with the Tea Diet. My mood has changed, my outlook on life is much more focused, and I am regaining the confidence I once had. I have realized how afraid of making changes I was. Now I feel great and more energized than I have in years. To be honest, I went from a tired person who was in debt, hated her job, and did not like what she saw in the mirror, to an energetic, motivated woman who loves being alive and is passionate about life.

I'm glad I lost weight, but more importantly, this whole experience has been inspiring for me because on a day-to-day basis, I've never felt so good.

As I mentioned, I am getting married. Like many brides, I bought a dress two sizes too small and said, "I'm going to make myself fit into this." After eight weeks on the Ultimate Tea Diet, I decided to try the dress on and see if it was still too small. The zipper went up, and my jaw dropped down. I'm very excited!

3

The Metabolics of Tea:
Tea's Secret Weight-Loss Ingredients

A merica is a land of contradictions. It seems that for every step forward we take, whether it be in politics or pop culture, we take at least three steps backward. Our country's obsession with weight and weight loss is no exception.

Approximately 65 percent of Americans are overweight, and an astonishing 30.5 percent are considered obese. At the same time, Americans spend about $40 billion a year on weight-loss products and services. Which means that as our bodies are getting heavier and heavier, our wallets are getting lighter and lighter chasing after that fad diet or magic pill that will bring us back to being trim, fit, and healthy.

Well, I am here to tell you that you can put your $40 billion back in your pocket and you can stop falling for those late-night infomercials that show you trumped-up before and after photos to try and make you believe that all you have to do is take three incredibly expensive pills a day and you'll lose hundreds of pounds and develop washboard abs as well. Who do they think they're kidding? Those supplements never work. Who knows what's really in them, and what harm they may be doing to your body and health?

That is what is so amazing about the Ultimate Tea Diet. If you follow the balanced meal plan in chapter 8, which includes my mantra, "Find the teas you love and drink them all day," you will lose weight. And because you are using no drugs or supplements to achieve your weight loss, you don't have to worry about reading any fine print. Drinking tea has no harmful side effects, which is why people have been drinking it for close to 5,000 years.

Tea3: Tea's Secret Weight-Loss Ingredients

Everyone and their mother knows that tea is good for you (you'll find out more about tea's amazing health benefits in the next chapter). Just think about when you were last ill. Did you say, "Hey honey, can you get me a cup of coffee?" No way! You said, "Hey honey, can you get me a cup of tea?" But only in the last ten years or so have scientists begun to turn their attention to the connection between drinking tea and losing weight. Turns out there are three incredible ingredients in tea that work synergistically to influence the metabolic and nervous systems to help take the weight off and keep it off.

Each one of these ingredients taken alone has a degree of efficiency in helping the body to shed pounds. But it's the combination—the mighty triumvirate I call "Tea3"—that gives tea its weight-loss wallop. And remember, these three ingredients are found naturally in the *Camellia sinensis* plant, not manufactured in a chemical plant. Tea is truly a miracle of nature—what I consider to be the most perfect plant ever created. I can't help but get passionate when I speak about tea because I get so caught up in just how much nature can provide for us, if we only let it.

And every day I get more and more excited about tea as one scientific study after another proves that my faith in Cami is justified, especially where tea and weight loss is concerned. There is hard science behind the tea–weight loss connection that explains the synergy of the Tea3 powerful ingredients: caffeine, L-theanine, and epigallocatechin-3-gallate (EGCG). The names may be tricky but the science isn't, and this chapter will explain what they are and how they work together to increase your metabolism, keep you feeling satiated, and give you more energy without setting your nerves on edge.

Secret Ingredient #1: Caffeine

It's difficult to separate Tea3's ingredients in terms of each one's influence on weight loss, since each has an effect on the other. But to help you understand how the overall process works, I'll give it a try in simple nonscientific terms, because I need things made simple for me to understand them and then incorporate them into my life.

Let's start with caffeine. Caffeine is a chemical found naturally in more than sixty species of plants, including coffee, tea, and cocoa. Mother Nature put caffeine in plants as a defense from insects consuming the leaves; caffeine is very bitter. Too much caffeine can be detrimental to your health, as you will find out in detail in chapter 10. However, caffeine is not all bad. It is a natural stimulant that has been shown to boost the process known as thermogenesis, or the generation of heat in the body. This process is at the center of weight loss; it is the way in which fat molecules are "burned." Thermal energy is divided into calories; the more energy that is expended, the more calories you will burn. Numerous studies have shown that caffeine increases energy expenditure.

A study published in the *American Journal of Clinical Nutrition* in 1989 concluded that "caffeine at commonly consumed doses can have a significant influence on energy balance and may promote thermogenesis in the treatment of obesity."

This is why you find caffeine in most of the over-the-counter diet supplements on supermarket and drugstore shelves today, many of which have extremely unhealthy side effects. In another study published in the *American Journal of Clinical Nutrition,* this one in 1999, scientists studying the use of green tea extracts concluded that tea not only promoted thermogenesis, but that unlike caffeine alone, which arouses your nervous system and speeds up your heartbeat, the use of green tea extract was "not accompanied by an increase in heart rate." To summarize these two studies, the consumption of tea will increase the burning of calories and promote weight loss without increasing your heart rate.

This leaves open the possibility of using green tea as an alternative to stimulant-based diet drugs found in the stores and advertised on TV, which may cause adverse effects on obese individuals and patients with hypertension (high blood pressure) and other cardiovascular conditions. Tea does not have these same adverse side effects because it has the next two secret ingredients: L-theanine and EGCG.

Secret Ingredient #2: L-Theanine

There is only one plant in the world (besides one obscure mushroom) that contains secret ingredient #2, and that plant is—you guessed it—*Camellia sinensis.* L-theanine (el-THEE-uh-neen) is a non-protein-based amino acid that constitutes between 1 and 2 percent of the dry weight of tea leaves. Caffeine makes up only about 0.5 percent.

As I said earlier, caffeine is a stimulant. It revs up many of your body's processes and sends your nervous system into a state of shock. After ingestion, it is secreted into the bloodstream and makes its way to the brain where it stimulates your beta brain waves (see TEAser box).

TEASER

Brain Waves

Brain waves are electrical impulses that correlate to different types of mental states and moods. There are four categories of brain waves:

- ❖ **Alpha:** predominantly present during states of relaxed alertness
- ❖ **Beta:** predominantly present during highly stressful or exciting situations
- ❖ **Delta:** predominantly present during the deepest stage of sleep
- ❖ **Theta:** predominantly present during light sleep and drowsiness

Beta brain waves are meant to be stimulated for the fight-or-flight response: when you are in danger, when you get into a car accident, when something happens to a member of your family. That's when your body needs to get stimulated, and you actually *want* to get into a state of stress. You want to be able to lift a car off your loved one, or run a 100-yard dash in ten seconds to get away from a mugger in the night.

But most of the time, we are not in situations that produce such intense states of excitement or stress, even though the caffeine rush is signaling so to the brain. This is why the L-theanine in tea is so important, and what makes Cami the most perfect plant. Several minutes after the caffeine has entered your system, the L-theanine is secreted from the small intestine into the blood system and into the brain where it stimulates alpha brain waves, which produce a state of relaxed and effortless alertness, thus canceling out the harmful effects of the caffeine. Since caffeine has already reached the brain and gotten a bit of a head start, so to speak, you will still get that short wake-up blast you want in the morning—but without the jitters and palpitations that come from other caffeinated beverages like coffee, the ubiquitous energy drinks, and cola. Now you begin to see why I love the Cami plant; caffeine is allowed into your system for the weight-loss benefits and stimulation, then shortly thereafter, L-theanine comes along to cancel out its harmful effects.

Because of L-theanine's effect on alpha brain waves, it is a natural medicine for the relief of stress, anxiety and tension. In fact, in 2004, researchers in Australia compared L-theanine to alprazolam (Xanax), a medication often prescribed to relieve anxiety. They found that L-theanine tended to reduce anxiety during a relaxation phase of the study, while the drug had no such effect.

Researchers have also found that L-theanine appears to play a role in the formation of gamma-aminobutyric acid (GABA), which blocks the release of the neurotransmitters dopamine and serotonin to promote a state of calm relaxation.

But that's not all. When stress levels decrease, so do levels of cortisol, a hormone that, when stimulated, increases appetite and influences where body fat will be stored (mainly in the abdominal region). In January 2007, scientists from the Department of Epidemiology and Public Health at the University College of London published findings on tea's effect on cortisol levels. The study, in the journal *Psychopharmacology,* found that people who drank tea were able to lower their stress levels faster than those who were given a placebo. For six weeks, participants drank either four cups of black tea a day, or four cups of a caffeinated placebo. After the six weeks, both groups were given two challenging behavioral tasks. Both groups were found to have similar stress levels when the tasks were completed; however, an hour later the cortisol levels had dropped by an average of 47 percent in the tea-drinking group compared with 27 percent in the caffeinated placebo group. So it seems that L-theanine not only reverses caffeine's harmful effects but assists to reduce stress, which in turn reduces appetite and the storage of fat in your body.

Secret Ingredient #3: EGCG

Even if you're not familiar with L-theanine, chances are you've heard of EGCG. It stands for a chemical compound called Epigallocatechin-3-gallate, and it's been appearing on a lot of highly visible labels lately. Bottled teas are now proudly announcing EGCG as an ingredient in their beverage (even though it's in *all* tea), and even the Coca-Cola company has jumped on the bandwagon with Enviga, a sparkling green tea beverage that contains EGCG and caffeine (and a host of artificial sweeteners and preservatives).

What is EGCG? It is a chemical compound known as a catechin, which is a subclass of polyphenols, compounds known for their antioxidant properties. Antioxidants are substances found in tea (and many other foods) that can prevent or slow the oxidative damage to the cells of the body. When the cells use oxygen, as they do all day, they naturally produce free radicals (by-products) which can cause damage to the cells. Antioxidants act as "free-radical policemen" and hence prevent and repair damage done by these free radicals. But EGCG is more than a potent antioxidant. In combination with Tea3's other secret ingredients, it is a potent factor in stimulating weight loss. Studies have shown that green tea extracts (containing EGCG) markedly inhibit enzymes in the pancreas that help to digest fat in vitro (meaning "in a test tube"), which may translate into reduced fat digestion in humans.

In a study appearing in 2005 in the *Journal of Clinical Nutrition,* thirty-eight Japanese men were each given a 340-milliliter bottle (roughly two cups) of oolong tea to drink with dinner each day. Half of the men got tea laced with about 22 milligrams of green tea catechins (mostly EGCG), and the rest got tea spiked with 960 milligrams of catechins.

All of the participants were put on a calorie-counting diet. After twelve weeks, both groups of men lost weight. Those drinking the low-catechins tea lost approximately 3 pounds, while the high-catechins group lost an average of more than 5 pounds. Most important, much of the weight loss in the second group came from fat—total fat volume fell 10.3 percent in the high-catechins group, while it fell only 2.6 percent in the others. Both groups found that they had lost inches off their waistlines.

The Ultimate Tea Diet TEAmmates all had the same result (although they lost an average of 12 pounds and 15.7 inches overall in eight weeks)! They all were proud to admit that their clothes were fitting better, and most were actually loose around the waist. *This is what is in store for you, too.*

Other reasons EGCG helps you lose weight include:

* *The Dynamic Duo: EGCG and Caffeine*: We've already learned that the caffeine in tea stimulates thermogenesis, the biochemical process by which fat in the body is burned to produce energy. Studies have now shown that there is a synergistic interaction between EGCG and caffeine that further promotes energy expenditure. A 1999 study in which a group of men were given 90 mg of EGCG three times daily concluded that the men taking the EGCG burned 266 more calories than those who were given placebos. The authors of the study concluded that EGCG not only stimulated but prolonged fat tissue thermogenesis to a much greater extent than just caffeine alone, and that tea's "thermogenic properties could reside primarily in an interaction between its high content in catechin-polyphenols and caffeine . . ." This proves that EGCG helps burn fat even if you're doing nothing other than sitting

around drinking tea all day. So the more tea you drink the more fat you burn.

* *EGCG and Triglycerides:* Triglycerides are a form of fat carried through the bloodstream in transporters called lipoproteins. The problem is that lipoproteins that have an abundance of triglycerides also have an abundance of cholesterol, which, as we know, can lead to heart disease. EGCG actually cleanses the blood of the additional triglycerides before they're deposited into the adipose (fat) tissue. In so doing, it's also lowering cholesterol levels. Now follow this closely because it is that important: if in fact the triglycerides are being cleansed by EGCG, your arteries and veins start to clear. If your arteries are clear, you're getting more oxygen into your blood, which gives you more energy, which in turn allows you to expend more energy and burn more calories and lose weight.

* *EGCG Reduces Insulin Production:* In a study on insulin published in the *Journal of Biological Chemistry* in April 2006, researchers found that EGCG could modulate insulin secretion by inhibiting glutamate dehydrogenase (GDH). GDH plays a dominant role in stimulating the secretion of insulin. Scientists studied the effects of EGCG on GDH and found that these compounds could inhibit GDH and therefore inhibit insulin secretion, which is good for weight loss.

Why are insulin levels so important for weight loss? Because insulin plays a major role in weight gain, and even keeps us from losing weight. The more insulin produced, the harder it is to lose weight. We get most of our energy from carbohydrates, which are digested and broken down into glucose, or blood sugar. When blood sugar levels rise, insulin, produced in the pancreas, begins to do its job, which is to escort blood sugar into the liver and muscles where it's turned into glycogen and waits to be burned as energy. If there's more blood sugar than there is cell storage space, the excess is converted into fat.

If you are consistently subjecting your cells to carbohydrate overload and your body is storing too much blood sugar as fat, the sensors that are normally receptive to insulin begin to shut down. The body continues to produce the insulin, but can no longer utilize it efficiently or effectively. So you have insulin being produced with no use other than telling your body to burn less fat and store more fat; this is commonly referred to as insulin resistance.

That begins a vicious cycle: When you are overweight, fat cells inhibit the release of glucose for energy because you have too much insulin. Because glucose is not being used for energy, it is locked into its storage space in the cell, and no more can get in. When more carbohydrates are consumed, and more glucose and insulin are produced, there is nowhere for them to go, so the glucose is turned into fat that in turn inhibits the use of glucose . . . It becomes harder and harder to lose weight because your body has become an automatic fat-producer. The more tea you drink, the lower the insulin level in your body.

✳ *Tea's EGCG enhances insulin's effectiveness:* In a study published in 2002 in the *Journal of Agricultural Food Chemistry,* black, green, and oolong teas (but not tisanes) were all shown to increase insulin activity (effectiveness) by more than 15 percent in vitro (test tube). The higher the insulin effectiveness (as caused by EGCG), the better your ability to convert sugars into energy, and the greater your ability to lose weight. The more tea you drink, the higher your insulin's effectiveness.

This is good news for people with type 2 diabetes (if you have diabetes, be sure to consult your physician before making any changes in your diet). Diabetes means that you either are not producing enough insulin, or that your cells are becoming insensitive to the insulin that is there. Since drinking tea makes insulin more effective, it may be able to prevent the disease, or at least to postpone its onset.

Put Them All Together . . .

In case you haven't already gotten the point, here's one more reason that the Tea3 combination is so effective in aiding weight loss:

* ✱ *Tea increases fat burning:* Another study, this one published in 2001 in the American Society for Nutritional Sciences' *Journal of Nutrition,* divided participants into four groups who, over a three-day period, consumed 1) water, 2) full-strength tea, 3) half-strength tea, and 4) water containing 270mg caffeine (equivalent to the concentration in the full-strength tea). Energy expenditure was significantly increased for both the full-strength tea and the caffeinated water treatments. In addition, fat oxidation (burning) was significantly higher (12 percent) when subjects consumed the full-strength tea rather than water, which shows us that caffeine alone is not as good as the Tea3's combination for losing weight.

It would be possible for me to go on and on, listing study after study that proves that drinking tea will help you lose weight, and you can find many of them listed in the reference section at the back of this book, or online. But it should be clear to you by now that there is solid scientific evidence to back up the claims of Tea3's weight-loss benefits. The beauty of this is that all you have to do to obtain these wonderful benefits and start dropping pounds and inches is to find the teas you love and start to drink them all day. Now doesn't that sound like something you can do? I know it does! It's easy and it works!

> *If you are cold, tea will warm you. If you are heated, it will cool you. If you are depressed, it will cheer you. If you are excited, it will calm you.*
> WILLIAM GLADSTONE, BRITISH PRIME MINISTER

TEAmmate Profile

Name: Christine A.
Age: 28
Total Weight Loss: 10.5
Total Inches Lost: 11.5
Favorite Tea: Dr. Tea's Candy Bar Black Tea

I have struggled with my weight for the past eight years and done the whole yo-yo dieting thing. Nothing was life-changing for me on those diets. I lost weight and gained it back because it never fit in my life. I was always craving something I couldn't have.

A little over a year ago I gained a lot of weight because I had broken my ankle on a hike. I was not allowed to exercise and so I got very depressed. Then, just when my ankle was healed I notice my whole leg was swollen and had it examined. I found out I had a blood clot and couldn't exercise for at least six months because of the medicine they had me on. I got more depressed and, of course, gained more weight. After nearly one year I finally received the okay to exercise from my doctor. I was on a mission to find the perfect plan for my life . . . a plan that would not just fit into my life but would become part of my life forever.

I planned on going to LA with my best girlfriends after we heard about Dr. Tea on TV. We knew we wanted to go by and meet him and try dr. tea's teas. The day I met him, I knew my life was going to change for the better. He told me about the Tea Diet.

I listened to Dr. Tea talk about all the benefits of drinking and cooking with tea and what it does to you, your body, and energy. He has been where I am today and knows exactly what I feel right now in my life about my weight. That was a big turning point for me and I knew I could do this . . . and *would* do this! What did I have to lose? I love tea and get to lose weight in the process. I knew this was the plan for me.

With the Ultimate Tea Diet plan you can have what you crave . . . in tea! I love french fries and guess what? He has a tea for that craving. I had to drink that tea a lot at lunch because I so badly wanted french fries, and it replaced that craving in my life. I also have a sweet tooth. Dr. Tea has some of the best sweet teas I could ever dream of. Every time I would feel my sweet tooth taking over, I would brew Dr. Tea's Candy Bar Tea and the craving would be satisfied! Now I crave the tea instead of the sweets! Whatever your craving, you can find a tea just right for you!

In just a week of being on the Ultimate Tea Diet, I had so much more energy I couldn't believe it. I was drinking tea all day long and felt the benefits Dr. Tea was talking about. My appetite was shrinking! I couldn't believe it! At times when I normally ate a lot, I ate a little and was full. What an amazing feeling. Even my husband was following the plan and seeing a change in his appetite and energy. I had enough energy to exercise, and wanted to! I started sleeping again at night without struggling to fall asleep! After a couple weeks, I started to see my clothes getting loose on me. I had a favorite pair of capris I haven't been able to wear in two years. I tried them on and they fit perfectly. I was amazed and was so proud of myself.

But the best thing happened one night when my husband asked me to go running around the block with him. I have struggled with asthma since high school and have the worst time running. I was a little nervous because I knew that I wouldn't make it around the block. I thought that after I passed four houses, I would have to walk. But I agreed to go anyway. We started to run and I was doing great. We passed that fourth house and I was still feeling great! I was now half way around the block and still going. My husband asked, "How you doing?" I said "Fine!!!" As we came around the last turn and I could see our house, I felt so good. As soon as we got to our driveway I started to cry! I was so impressed with myself, I knew then I was on the right track to getting healthy!

As each week passes I see changes in my body in different ways. My tummy looks less and less like I'm pregnant and my legs look less and less like cottage cheese. My acne is clearing up, my eating habits have changed—I don't want the junk food or french fries anymore. My stress has leveled out as well. I feel so much more confident about myself. I walk with my head up because I don't have a reason anymore to feel depressed or upset with my life.

There is nothing more exciting than knowing I'm on the right track to taking back control of *my* life! If I can do it . . . so can you!

4

Tea's Other Health Benefits

Imagine that you are a research scientist scanning the earth's flora and fauna, looking for those natural substances that might help the human race ward off disease and maintain healthy bodies. Imagine that you are looking for foods that could help prevent cancer, heart disease, osteoporosis, Alzheimer's, and stroke; that could lower blood pressure, reduce weight, decrease inflammation, protect against wrinkles and sun damage; and that could increase creativity and peak performance.

Now imagine that you found all of those properties in one inexpensive, noncaloric, readily available, good-tasting natural plant-derived substance.

You would be just like me; ecstatic, excited, over-the-moon, and anxious to spread to the waiting world word of your fantastic new discovery: tea.

Of course, you would soon realize that your "new" discovery was more than 4,700 years old—but it wasn't until the last century that scientists began to truly understand just how many rich and varied benefits there are in each and every cup of tea.

* * *

So now it's time for a short, but important, science lesson. Please, do not be put off by this. I'm including this information so that you will understand and appreciate all of tea's incredible health benefits. Take the time to read this chapter so that you too will come to understand what I have been reading about and analyzing for the past fifteen years, about what this miracle plant can do for us above and beyond weight loss. Remember, as we learned in chapter 1, all tea comes from the same plant, so even though the medical studies below only used one type of tea, all of the other types of tea would produce similar results.

Of Flavonoids and Free Radicals

What is it about tea that makes it so healthy? It begins with free radicals. A free radical is an oxygen molecule with an odd number of electrons in the outer ring of one of its atoms. Free radicals are unstable because of their missing electrons. To try to correct this condition, free radicals grab on to healthy cells and try to "steal" their electrons. What results, however, is that more free radicals are created, causing a chain reaction with the potential of causing a tremendous amount of cellular destruction. Over time, free radical activity can produce some extremely damaged, and in some instances, malignant (cancerous) cells.

Free radicals are produced naturally as oxygen interacts with organic matter (cut into an apple, leave it out on the counter and it turns brown—that is oxidation). Our bodies are constantly oxidizing. Sadly, we help the process along when we eat foods that have been refined and processed or fried in fats and oils at superhigh heat. Our bodies are not designed to cope with so much free radical buildup. Once we go past that threshold, our cells begin to age prematurely, and we contribute to our own journey towards disease and disability.

We would have no hope at all if it wasn't for antioxidants; they come to the rescue by destroying free radicals and slowing down the oxidation process. Turns out tea is rich in antioxidants called flavonoids, EGCG being one of the most potent ones (EGCG is a catechin, a subclass of polyphenols, which is in turn a subclass of flavonoids).

White tea has the largest amount of these flavonoids, then green, then oolong, then black. For the purposes of the Ultimate Tea Diet, it really does not matter which tea you are drinking because the differences in the amounts of flavonoids are small.

According to the Department of Food Science and Human Nutrition of Iowa State University, there are about 316 milligrams of flavonoids in a cup of green tea; a cup of black tea contains about 268 milligrams of flavonoids. Scientists have calculated that the tea plant ranks as one of the highest in total flavonoid content. The Agricultural Research Service, a branch of the United States Department of Agriculture, states that "green tea contains more simple flavonoids, called catechins, while black tea contains more complex varieties, called thearubigins and theaflavins. Some polyphenols have recently been determined—in test tube studies—to be more potent antioxidants than the well-known vitamins A, C, and E." Research has shown that both catechins and theaflavins are equally effective in scavenging free radicals and keeping you in good health.

TEASER

Free Radicals and Exercise: Good News and Bad News

The bad news is that exercise, which we all know is critical to weight loss, actually generates free radicals.

But don't let that stop you from your morning run, power walk, or resistance training! The good news is that if you drink a cup of tea before you exercise, you are not only pumping iron, you are pumping antioxidants into your bloodstream and fending off the oxidative damage caused to the cells.

In fact, some scientists believe that tea is even healthier than water. In August 2006, the *European Journal of Clinical Nutrition* published a review of tea-based studies conducted between 1990 and 2004 that reached some fascinating conclusions:

* Tea is not dehydrating. Very high doses of caffeine are dehydrating—but a cup of tea, even very strong tea, has nowhere near the amount of caffeine necessary to dehydrate the body. So go ahead and fill up your water bottles with tea and see and feel the difference as Dr. Carrie Ruxton explains below.

* Green tea is not healthier than black tea. Both types of tea contain similar amounts of antioxidants, although they are of different types. They both provide the same health benefits.

* Drinking three or more cups of tea a day (three cups equals 24 ounces) can reduce the risk of a wide range of health problems, ranging from cancer to heart disease.

Dr. Ruxton, lead author of the study, told the BBC News that she recommends 1.5 to 2 litres (six to eight cups, or 48 to 64 ounces) of fluid intake a day, and, she says, "that can include tea." And, perhaps most important, she told the BBC, *"Drinking tea is actually better for you than drinking water. Water is essentially replacing fluid. Tea replaces fluid and contains antioxidants so it's got two things going for it."*

Of Inflammation and Immunity

Another good reason for drinking tea is that it boosts your immune system, a complex set of organs, tissues, and specialized cells that protects the body from bacteria, viruses, and other internal and external toxins. When these toxins invade the body, they trigger an inflammatory response. Injured tissue releases chemicals that cause swelling in order to isolate the "invader" from further contact with the body. However, when the immune system encounters unusually large amounts of toxins, other symptoms are added to the swelling, such as redness, stiffness, and pain, and diseases including asthma, rheumatoid arthritis, allergies, and many other serious autoimmune maladies can occur.

Several recent studies have shown that both L-theanine and EGCG are effective in boosting the immune system and in fighting inflammation. In one study, published in 2003 in the *Proceedings of the National Academy of Sciences*, Harvard scientists found that tea acts as a sort of natural vaccine that "teaches" immune cells to recognize markers on the surface of invading toxins. Prior to the study, participants were measured for certain T cells that play a crucial role in resisting infection. Then they were asked to drink five or six cups a day of either tea or coffee for four weeks. When they were subsequently measured, the tea drinkers—*but not the coffee drinkers*—saw increased production of an important disease-fighting protein on their T cells. The researchers concluded that the L-theanine in tea helps "prime human . . . T-cells . . . [to] provide natural resistance to microbial infections."

Other studies have shown that EGCG helps block production of a key molecule (interleukin-8) that causes inflammation in many conditions like arthritis. A study involving arthritis-prone mice showed that when they were given the human equivalent of four cups of green tea a day, they halved their risk of developing the disease. A 2007 study from the University of Michigan found that EGCG inhibited the production of several molecules in the immune system that contribute to inflammation and joint damage in people with rheumatoid arthritis. And in another 2007 study, Dr. Stephen Hsu, a cell biologist in the Medical College of Georgia's Department of Oral Biology and Maxillofacial Pathology, investigated Sjogren's syndrome, an autoimmune disease that damages the glands that produce saliva and causes what is commonly known as dry mouth. He noted that about 30 percent of elderly Americans suffer from dry mouth, while only 5 percent of the elderly in China, where tea is widely consumed, suffer from the problem. Some participants were given green tea to drink, and others were given water. At the end of the study, the green tea group showed significantly less damage to their salivary glands. Dr. Hsu stated that these results reinforced earlier findings that showed a similar phenomenon in a petri dish, and that further study could help determine tea's protective role in other autoimmune diseases.

Matters of the Heart

In the late 1960s, American scientists noticed some interesting findings. While doing autopsies, they observed that the arteries of tea-drinking Chinese Americans had only two-thirds as much coronary artery disease as Caucasian coffee drinkers. Since that time, many more studies have shown a link between drinking tea and preventing heart disease. As we learned in the last chapter, tea helps to cleanse the blood of triglycerides and cholesterol. In 2003, the *Archives of Internal Medicine* published a study in which, over a twelve-week period, 240 Chinese men and women with moderately high cholesterol were given either a green tea extract augmented with theaflavins from black tea or a placebo with no tea. After the twelve weeks, the placebo group had no changes in their total cholesterol or their "bad" LDL cholesterol levels. In the tea group, however, total cholesterol dropped by 11.3 percent and LDL by 16.4 percent. At the same time, the "good" HDL cholesterol levels increased by 2.3 percent in the tea-drinking group, while the placebo group saw an increase of only 0.7 percent.

Another study, published in 2003, using black tea, found a 6- to 10-percent reduction in blood lipids (fats) in black tea drinkers in just three weeks. The Agricultural Research Service reported the study's authors' conclusion: "Drinking black tea, in combination with following a prudent diet moderately low in fat, cholesterol, and saturated fatty acids, reduces total and LDL cholesterol by significant amounts and may reduce the risk of coronary heart disease."

Tea also protects the heart by helping to lower blood pressure. Hypertension, or high blood pressure, is the most common form of heart disease, and is a major risk factor for heart-related death. A study of Chinese tea drinkers published in 2004 showed that drinking as little as a half-cup of green or oolong tea per day may lower the risk of high blood pressure by nearly 50 percent. Researchers found that men and women who drank tea on a daily basis for at least a year were much less likely to develop hypertension than those who didn't, and the more tea they drank, the bigger the benefits. Those who drank at least a half-cup of moderate strength green or oolong tea per day for a year had a 46-percent lower risk of developing hypertension than those who didn't drink tea. Among those who drank more than two and a half cups of tea per day, the risk of high blood pressure was reduced by 65 percent.

Tea and the Big C

The evidence that tea helps prevent cancer is overwhelming. Since the 1990s, hundreds of studies have been performed showing that tea can inhibit the formation of tumors, and slow the growth of those already formed. In 1997, researchers at the University of Kansas discovered that the antioxidant power of EGCG is about 100 times greater than vitamin C and twenty-five times greater than vitamin E in protecting DNA from the kind of free radical damage that is thought to increase the risk of cancer. Researchers also found that EGCG is able to signal cancer cells to stop reproducing by promoting apoptosis, a normal cellular process leading to the death of a cell—without harming any healthy cells. One study out of Purdue University in 1998 found that an enzyme called quinol oxidase, or NOX, is necessary for the growth of both normal and cancerous cells. The overactive form of NOX is known as tNOX, for tumor-associated NOX. In test tubes, using purified NOX protein solutions, researchers found that low doses of EGCG—such as those that could be consumed by drinking several cups of tea a day—were capable of inhibiting the activity of the tNOX cells but did not inhibit the NOX activity of healthy cells.

Here are just a few examples of what cancer-related studies have shown:

* *Tea and breast cancer*: Scientists have long noted that breast cancer is much less common in countries where green tea is regularly consumed. One Japanese study found a decreased risk of recurrence for early-stage cancer patients who drank three or more cups of green tea. This suggests at least the possibility that regular green tea consumption may help prevent recurrence of breast cancer in early-stage cases. A Chinese study found that women who consumed at least 26 ounces of green tea leaves each year had a 39-percent reduced risk of breast cancer compared

to nondrinkers. Twenty-six ounces of dried leaves per year equates to only 300 cups of green tea over the course of a year, which equals less than one cup per day.

✳ *Tea and ovarian cancer:* A Swedish study of more than 61,000 women, published in 2005, showed that women who consumed two or more cups of green or black tea every day lowered their risk for ovarian cancer by 46 percent, with each additional cup of tea lowering the risk by another 18 percent. A study of 1,200 American women, published in 2007, showed that the more black tea the women drank, the greater protection against ovarian cancer: compared to women who did not drink black tea, women with a usual consumption of at least two cups a day experienced a 30-percent decline in ovarian cancer risk.

✳ *Tea and lung cancer:* A study published in 2003 found that smokers who drank four cups of decaffeinated green tea per day demonstrated a 31-percent decrease in biomarkers of oxidative DNA damage in white blood cells as compared to those who drank four cups of water. Oxidative DNA damage is implicated in the development of various forms of cancer. A study published in 2007 in the *Journal of Inflammation* found that black tea had a positive preventive effect. In this study, guinea pigs were subjected to cigarette smoke exposure and then given water or black tea to drink. The cigarette smoke, needless to say, caused damage to the guinea pigs' lungs, which was prevented when they were given black tea infusions to drink instead of water.

✳ *Tea and prostate cancer:* Other than skin cancer, prostate cancer is the most common cancer affecting men. More than 230,000 American men are diagnosed with this disease each year, according to the American Cancer Society. A study published in the December 1, 2004 issue of *Cancer Research* showed that the polyphenols present in green tea help prevent the spread of prostate cancer by targeting molecular pathways that shut down the proliferation and spread of tumor cells, as well as inhibiting the growth of tumor-nurturing blood vessels. An Italian study published in 2005 found that a supplement containing antioxidants from green tea was 90 percent effective in preventing prostate cancer in men at high risk for the disease. That study found that after a year of taking green tea catechins, only one man in a group of thirty-two who were at higher risk of prostate cancer actually developed the disease, while nine men in a group of thirty high-risk men who took a placebo without tea developed prostate cancer.

Whether you choose to follow the Ultimate Tea Diet or not, it's a good idea to lose weight if you want to avoid prostate cancer. An American Cancer Society study that included 900,000 Americans who were followed over sixteen years showed that the increased risk of prostate cancer for men who were overweight was 8 percent, for obese men the risk was increased by 20 percent, and severely obese men were more than 34 percent times more likely than men of normal weight to suffer from the disease.

A study of Australian men reported that obese men were 2.2 times more likely to develop aggressive prostate cancer than lean men, with each 22 pounds of excess weight boosting the risk by 40 percent. And abdominal obesity has been linked to nearly a threefold increase in the risk of clinical prostate cancer in China.

* *Tea and other cancers*: Hundreds of other studies have been done showing that tea can help prevent many other types of cancer, including skin, stomach, bladder, and colon cancers.

* *Tea and chemotherapy*: Preliminary studies have shown that L-theanine enhances the results of some chemotherapy drugs by preventing cancerous cells from rejecting the drugs after the drugs have entered the tumor cells. L-theanine has also been shown to ameliorate some of the side effects of these drugs.

TEASER

Like Red Meat? Have Some Tea

Did you know that powerful mutagens (compounds known to cause cancer) form when you broil or fry meat? Scientists believe that these mutagens increase the risk of both breast and colon cancer. So do you have to give up your favorite protein?

No way! A study published in the journal *Mutation Research* in 2002 showed that the application of green tea and black tea to both surfaces of beef before cooking inhibits the formation of the mutagens. So go to chapter 11 and experiment with the tea rub recipes you'll find there. Find the one(s) you like and rub on that tea—and be generous. The more tea you rub on, the fewer cancer-causing agents in your beef. And, oh yes—the tastier your beef!

The accumulated evidence showing tea as a preventative agent against cancer is so strong, it prompted researchers from the Radiation Effects Research Foundation in Hiroshima, Japan to state that "daily consumption of green tea in sufficient amounts will help to prolong life by avoiding premature death, particularly death caused by cancer." Although this study used only green tea, we now know that all true tea will confer the same benefits.

Brain TEAsers

If you are in the middle of an artistic endeavor, trying to solve a complicated problem, or about to enter an athletic event, you might want to take a short break and have a nice cup of tea. When the L-theanine in your tea of choice stimulates your alpha brain waves, it generates a state of relaxed alertness—and it also enhances your ability to concentrate while it promotes mental clarity. It improves your ability to learn new things. Increased activity in alpha brain waves leads to heightened creativity. And sports scientists have shown that increases in alpha brain waves usually precede peak performance. So if you want to be your best and do your best, it seems that a cup of tea just might be your best bet!

And that goes for protecting your brain as well. A Japanese study of approximately 6,000 women found that those who drank five or more cups of green tea a day were significantly less likely than those who drank no tea to suffer a stroke or a cerebral hemorrhage. A Dutch study in the *Archives of Internal Medicine* in 1996 revealed that drinking five cups of black tea per day also reduced the likelihood of stroke—by as much as 69 percent.

And in 2004, an English team determined that both green and black tea inhibited the activity of enzymes associated with the development of Alzheimer's disease, but that coffee had no significant effect. Although there are drugs currently on the market that serve the same purpose, they often have unpleasant side effects. Lead researcher Dr. Ed Okello, who is a lecturer with Newcastle University's School of Biology, said: "Although there is no cure for Alzheimer's, tea could potentially be another weapon in the armory which is used to treat this disease and slow down its development."

Tea from the Outside In

While tea is performing all of its medical miracles on the inside of your body, it's improving the outside as well. In 2006, a team of American and German researchers published the results of their study of the effect of topically applied tea extracts on skin damage from radiation treatment in cancer patients. They found that the tea reduced the duration of skin damage by five to ten days, and concluded that the tea works at a cellular level to inhibit inflammatory pathways and reduce inflammation. Dr. Stephen Hsu, introduced earlier in this chapter, has conducted a number of studies on green tea and EGCG. In 2003, he and his colleagues published the findings of their study of the normal growth of skin cells versus the growth of the cells when exposed to EGCG. He was astonished to find that EGCG reactivated dying skin cells. In a news release from the Medical College of Georgia, Dr. Hsu said that "when exposed to EGCG, the old cells found in the upper layers of the epidermis appear to start dividing again. They make DNA and produce more energy." He also found that EGCG could benefit skin conditions from psoriasis to wrinkles and wounds. "If we can spur the skin cells to differentiate and proliferate," he said, "we can potentially accelerate the wound-healing process and prevent scarring."

More and more dermatologists are using tea-based products for their patients. Dr. Julia Tatum Hunter of Skin Fitness Plus in Beverly Hills recommends several of these products, as well as advising that her patients drink at least three cups of tea a day. "In today's toxic world where the ozone has been depleted, where the ultraviolet radiation induces increasingly more toxicity and inflammation in the skin, it's imperative to consume more antioxidants," says Dr. Hunter. "Tea not only tastes good, it can replace the soda and coffee that increase your toxicity and your inflammation. Inflammation affects the breakdown of collagen, which is what gives you wrinkles and causes your skin to sag as you get older. So the more tea you drink the better."

TEASER

Does Tea Stain Your Teeth?

The answer is: it might. Tea, along with coffee, cola, red wine, and grape juice, contains tannins, compounds that give these beverages their astringent qualities. These beverages are also known as "chromogenic," meaning that they have the ability, over time, to stain the teeth. A simple rule of thumb is that if a food or beverage can leave a permanent stain on clothes or carpets, it can probably stain your teeth as well. But teeth are very individual substances; some people's teeth can become discolored by these beverages, while others suffer no effects at all.

Here are some tips to follow if your teeth are changing color:

❖ Visit your dentist. Teeth naturally darken with age, so it may have nothing to do with what you eat or drink. There can also be pathological reasons for discoloration (like tooth decay), which only a dentist can identify. Be sure to go for regular cleanings, which can often take care of the staining problem.

❖ If you're drinking a lot of tea, rinse your mouth with plain water several times during the day.

❖ Brush often. Electric toothbrushes may be more effective at getting rid of staining than manual brushing.

❖ Floss regularly. Teeth often stain worse around the edges. That's where plaque builds up, and plaque attracts stain.

❖ Try drinking iced tea. Hot liquids penetrate tooth enamel more easily than cold. And it's even better if you drink your cold beverages through a straw, as you reduce the teeth's exposure to the staining beverages.

❖ Whiten your teeth. Your dentist may perform in-office bleaching, or you can try over-the-counter whitening strips, gels, or toothpastes. When selecting a whitener, be sure to look for the American Dental Association Seal of Acceptance, which assures that the product has met the ADA's standards of safety and effectiveness.

On a tooth-healthy note: Tea is a rich source of fluoride. Fluoride is a natural element found in the earth's crust as well as in water and air. It works with saliva to protect tooth enamel from plaque and sugars. The tea plant (Camellia sinensis) extracts fluoride from the soil, which then accumulates in its leaves. So tea, while it may cause some discoloration, is actually good for your teeth!

*   *   *

As with the previous chapter, I could go on and on about the benefits of tea. I haven't even covered all the areas of research; recent findings are showing that tea can help prevent osteoporosis and even, in preliminary studies, reduce the risk of HIV infection. With all of the studies mentioned above and the thousands more going on today, it is important to note that, unlike some other caffeinated drinks I know of (coffee, energy drinks, and sodas), there do not seem to be any down sides to drinking tea. There are no studies showing that tea does a body any harm. All the news about tea is good.

Now that you know all the incredible things tea can do for you, and now that you've started drinking tea (I hope), you're ready to start making important changes in your life. So go ahead and make yourself another cup of your favorite tea and let's begin the Ultimate Tea Diet.

Seven bowls of tea bring seven advantages:
one, it promotes the production of body fluids and quenches thirst;
two, it refreshes the mind;
three, it helps digestion;
four, it induces sweating to relieve the common cold;
five, it helps fat people reduce weight;
six, it activates thinking and strengthens memory;
and seven, it ensures longevity."

FROM *HEALTH BENEFITS OF TEA* BY LU TONG,
WRITTEN DURING THE TANG DYNASTY OVER 1,100 YEARS AGO

TEAmmate Profile

Name: Canary G.

Age: 52

Total Weight Loss: 19

Total Inches Lost: 26.5

Favorite Tea: Dr. Tea's Candy Bar Black Tea

When I walked into dr. tea's March 10, 2007, I had no idea my life was about to totally change. I didn't know I was about to discover something that would be so consuming and cause me to get so excited. I've been trying to lose weight for over ten years—sad to say, but it's true. I've tried everything, every diet, and nothing worked. Or if it did it was only for a minute, then I would lose interest and I always gained the weight back.

Since I've been on the Ultimate Tea Diet, something is very different for me this time. I was so ready to try something that would work, something I would believe in and something that would restore something that was very lost in me. Well, I found it, and it has continued daily to call my name.

What really sparked my interest in tea was a friend in South Carolina who told me she had lost 15 pounds in less than two months drinking green tea. A delivery man on my job told me how much better he felt drinking black tea and that I should try it. I thought to myself, I grew up drinking iced tea daily and maybe I should go back to my roots. I had a bag of green tea at the office and began to drink it daily for about two weeks. During those weeks I surfed the Net and kept reading about how tea promotes weight-loss.

While I was searching the internet, I went to Dr. Tea's website, talked with Dr. Tea and days later I visited dr. tea's. I sat at the bar, watched, listened, and drank the best-tasting tea I ever had in my life. People kept coming in one after another giving their testimonies about how great they felt, how much energy they now had, and how much weight they had lost.

The Ultimate Tea Diet is a program that is life changing—it can totally change your lifestyle, the way you think, the way you feel and how you look. The first week I lost 6.5 pounds and was totally blown away. I replaced coffee and sodas with eight to thirteen cups of tea a day. I found wonderful tasting flavored teas from dr. tea's such as Dr. Tea's Candy Bar Black Tea, White Blueberry, and Key Lime Pie Sherbet, just to name a few. It's almost like cheating in a good way to good health.

The Ultimate Tea Diet works naturally with your system and will cause changes you won't believe. My skin is clearer. I've lost inches all over my body and my exercising endurance has increased. I drink some of the trigger teas to curb my appetite for things such as candy bars, chips, and wine. Don't get me wrong, you will have those urges but they won't be as strong when drinking the teas.

You will learn how to eat healthy following the 14-day menu plan. You will learn how to adjust foods to your liking in a healthy way. I know you might be thinking, I can't eat this and I don't like that. This is where the teas come in. The teas taste so good to me that they gave me the motivation to change what I ate and the way it was prepared. I didn't think I ate that badly or anything, but I found a better way. Some of the recipes served as a guideline to get me off to a good start. I now find myself using tea in almost everything I cook—peas, cabbage, steak, eggs, you name it.

Most of all I changed my mind, I changed my way of thinking. "If I say I can, I will; if I say I can't, I won't." This program can and will work for anyone who would like to lose weight. You can lose at your own pace and you don't have to starve yourself or skip meals. The weight loss is amazing; you'll say, "Oh, I can do this." Everywhere I go it's me and my tea. I love it!

I am amazed at the results I've had being on the Ultimate Tea Diet. I am happy to say that my blood pressure medication has been cut in half. My clothes are loose-fitting and inches are melting away, oh happy day! I work out three to five times a week, I eat tasty foods that are good for me. I must say I have worked this Ultimate Tea Diet and it has worked me.

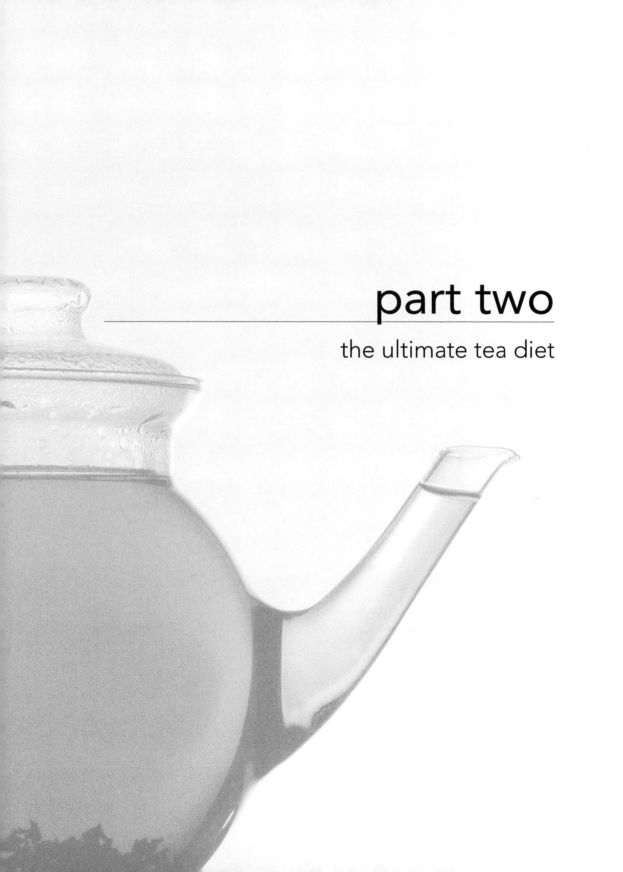

part two

the ultimate tea diet

The Tao of Tea:

You Can If You Think You Can

W hen you go on a diet, or start a new exercise plan, or stop drinking coffee, energy drinks, or diet soda, or want to change any bad habit in your life, you're asking a lot of yourself. Change is hard. No matter how much tea you drink, losing weight will be a temporary fix unless you address the way you think about your life and yourself. I didn't set out to write *The Ultimate Tea Diet* fifteen years ago when I made my life's turn. All I knew was that I had to make a change in my life. I had to get strong, I had to get healthy. I had to start changing who I was. I had to start changing how I thought about who I was.

When tea found me, it changed my life and my health, and it will change yours, too! I am my own best testimonial. You will read about my life-changing event, when I was 38, when I had to make a choice of staying on the same old road, going to the same old places, and feeling the same old way about who I was—or getting off that old road and making a turn onto a new one, a road of good health and good thought, with different sights and a completely different destination—a destination filled with great health and the energy of a man half my age. I made that turn. I had to! Isn't it time for you to make your turn, too?

At first, I had to crawl down that new road. Then I began walking, then jogging, running, and finally I was able to drive down that new road because I took control of my life. And, to my own amazement, I found that at every new turn there was tea or something to do with tea. I created the Ultimate Tea Diet (although it had no name at the time). I started by replacing one of the many cups of coffee I was drinking each day with one cup of tea instead; slowly I built up to as much tea as I could drink all day. I learned to cook with tea and noticed the difference in my physiology and my psychology almost immediately. I was much less frenetic. I was not so needy. I cut way down on the amount of alcohol I was drinking, and when I did drink I learned to make drinks with tea in them. I began to lose weight. I began to work out and to feel healthier and happier than ever before. I even began to meditate.

TEASER

Tea and Alcohol

I'm not encouraging anyone to drink alcohol. But if you do, I am encouraging you to drink tea before and after. That's because several animal studies have shown that the antioxidants in tea protect against liver and brain damage caused by alcohol.

In a study published in the January 2004 issue of the journal *Alcohol*, in which laboratory animals (okay—rats) were chronically intoxicated with alcohol for four weeks, green tea prevented damage to their livers. Another study, also published in 2004 in the journal *Food and Chemical Toxicology*, again involving intoxicated lab animals, looked at the effects of black tea and concluded: "These results indicated beneficial antioxidant effect of black tea regarding all examined tissue, but especially the liver." And other studies have shown that tea protects brain tissue against the free radical damage caused by alcohol consumption.

Now, please don't think I'm starting a Cult of Tea. You're not going to start begging barefoot, asking strangers for money for a cup of oolong. You're not going to give up your worldly possessions and go live with a houseful of other tea drinkers (unless you choose to). But if you want the Ultimate Tea Diet to be successful for you, you are going to have to make some changes.

My Story

When I was a young man of 18, I traveled to Europe for the first time. I had no money to speak of, so I rationed everything. My friends with more funds ate freely, while I sat there starving. At times the only thing I could afford was something to drink. I soon came to realize that the cappuccinos and espressos only added to my hunger. Drinking tea actually reduced my hunger pangs. I didn't know any of the scientific reasons for this that I later learned; I only knew that I didn't need as much food as I thought I did, all because I was drinking tea. Tea became my solace and my savior. It never failed to ease my hunger.

On the same trip, I remember that when I did have some food to eat, I made sure to give away a portion of my food to another. This act actually suppressed my appetite. I was more satisfied with what I had in front of me by giving a part of it away, and was not as hungry so soon thereafter. It is one of the unwritten laws of the universe.

After a while, I came home to my old life—and my old habits. I forgot about tea. I drank coffee all day. I ate sweets. I worked too much and played too hard. Life happened, and some of it was very painful. And then, when things were at their worst, I found my way back to tea.

When I was 38 years old, anyone who didn't know me (and even most who did) would look at me and think, "That guy has it all." In some ways I did. True, I had had a failed marriage and a bitter divorce. But I was very successful in business, first as a sports agent and then in the real estate field. True, my business life was not satisfying to me. I was addicted to coffee; I drank ten, twelve, fourteen cups of coffee a day. I had to have my fix every single day. But I had a multimillion-dollar four-story beach house in Malibu (where all the movie stars live). I had a hot, head-turning Ferrari. I traveled the world. I ate at the best tables at the best restaurants, partied with A-list crowd, dated women I didn't necessarily like, but who looked great on my arm. The truth was, I did have it all.

Almost. I didn't have *me*. Sounds corny, I know, and you've heard it over and over again. But one day as I was drinking my fourth or fifth morning coffee, standing alone on the fourth-floor deck in my beautiful beach house, just me and my dogs, I realized how empty it really was. How empty I was. And I was ready to end it all! A small jump four stories to the rocks and ocean below would have done very nicely.

I was an unhappy, moderately overweight, out-of-shape man who took a lot from life and gave back too little. But there was some voice inside of me that said, "Not today, Mark. You can get over this. You have to because there is something you still have to do."

Fifteen years ago, when I made that turn in my life's intersection, I made the conscious choice to change my life, and everything else changed. What changed first was the realization that my life to date was nothing more than the summation of all of my realities. I was what I had created for myself. I had created success in business, but I had also created an unsuccessful marriage. I had created a fabulous home for myself, but I had also created a lifestyle that was making me miserable. I had to change my reality to change my life.

I started to take a long look at *me*. I realized that I was going in the same direction, to the same old places, with the same old people, and with the same old results: unhappiness and disappointment. All the while I was hiding away, not wanting to be noticed, trying to blend into the background and be like everyone else. But I was living a lie. I really wanted to be noticed. I wanted to be in the limelight. I was crying out without saying a word, "PLEASE NOTICE ME! HERE I AM! I NEED YOUR HELP!"

But the only help that ever showed up was *me*.

I asked what I could do to help myself. What changes could I make in my behavior that could change my reality? One of the first things I looked at was how much coffee I was drinking, and what it was doing to me. I saw that I wasn't a great human being on coffee. I was on edge, I was treating people badly, I was flippant, tight, intense (and not in a good way). Without knowing why, I knew it was a negative influence in my life. So I started drinking tea.

Not because of its medicinal properties—I had no idea they existed. Not because it was a weight-loss aid—at the time, no one had ever suggested such a thing. Not because my family used to be in the tea business—the thought never crossed my mind. And certainly not because of the taste—I didn't even like the tea I was drinking at the time.

I started drinking tea because it was a hot beverage that seemed to me the closest thing I could get to coffee. I could put it in a coffee mug, drink several cups a day, and hope that it would help me fill the space that giving up coffee was leaving in my life. It was as if I had been a smoker and had started chewing gum to help wean me off the cigarettes.

Slowly, I began to realize that the tea was changing me. I started to want more tea, and better tea. I wanted to understand what was really happening to my mind and body. I began to read everything I could find about tea. I interviewed anyone available who knew anything about tea, from traditional doctors to homeopaths to naturalists and pathologists, and asked them to explain tea's special qualities. I traveled to all of the major tea producing regions of the world and learned directly from tea masters about producing teas and how to determine good from great teas. I went to tea auctions to witness firsthand what grades of tea companies were buying. I consulted with my father about our family's 200-year history in the tea business. I drank in every bit of information, just as I drank in my new beverage of choice, tea. I came to realize, not only from the changes in my life and body, that I was onto something that had to be shared with the rest of our country, that tea, combined with this proven diet, will be what's finally needed to wake up America to take a step towards good health one cup of tea at a time!

Although tea has been around for thousands of years, there has never been a face and voice of tea until tea found me and I found dr. tea's.

How "Dr. Tea" Came to Be

When my wife and I opened dr. tea's, we decided that my staff and I should wear lab coats so that we looked professional. We chose the orange color because it's the one the Dalai Lama wears, and he represents peace and tranquility.

One day, a group of six-year-olds was having a party at dr. tea's. One of them piped up and said, innocently enough, "Hey mommy, that guy in the orange coat sounds like a doctor." And that's how "Dr. Tea" was born.

Before I found tea, I had always been a behind-the-scenes person. I had never spoken out about anything in my life, much less written a book, appeared on television and radio, or been interviewed for magazines. But now I have this newly found voice and I am speaking out about tea to anyone who will listen. You can always pick me out in a crowd wherever I go, clad in my orange coat. I guess I am a perfect example of how you can change your life at any age if you are open to it!

The Ultimate Tea Diet is nothing more than my life's diet for the past fifteen years. The tea changed me. The L-theanine from the tea changed me. The polyphenols changed me. As a result, I was able to change my diet. I was able to start to meditate. I began exercising. I was able to let go of the negative influences in my life and began attracting kind, sensitive, positive people towards me, like my wonderful wife Julie.

The same thing can happen to you. But *you* have to be the one to make the changes. Of course, you will receive support and encouragement from friends and loved ones. But they cannot make changes for you. In the end, it is up to you. And the Ultimate Tea Diet is *all* about you; and that's why it works.

You Are the Driver; Tea Is the Vehicle

I had enough of the world I had created for myself. It was time to create some new realities and change my life. I did it, and boy, am I glad I did!

Tea was the vehicle to my new me but it was not everything I did or had to do. I began by figuring out what areas of *me* I needed and wanted to strengthen that would allow me to be happy and in control of the entire *me*. I decided to strengthen my mind, body, and soul.

I'm sure you've probably heard this before, people telling you to change this, that, or the other, and you've resisted. We all resist change; it's in our nature. I'm not telling you to do anything. I'm just letting you know what

I did and what worked for me. If one thing I say resonates with you, give it a try. Give yourself a chance. The only one who is going to benefit here is *you*!

This is what I did. I began by writing out the areas I was most concerned about along with a possible solution:

1. Problem: *Caffeine Addiction.* I needed help in ridding myself of my twelve- to fifteen-cup-a-day caffeine-from-coffee addiction.
   Possible Solution: Begin trading tea for coffee. Without the changes I made in the entire *me,* my addiction would have lasted longer than anticipated, or even worse, I may have returned to my old caffeine-from-coffee days and the old me. In addition to drinking tea, I began to work on the next three problems.

2. Problem: *Mind.* I needed help strengthening my mind to handle all of life's adversities and the ways I thought about myself.
   Possible Solution: Learn to retrain my mind by living by this mantra: *If I think and say I can, I will! If I think and say I can't, I won't!*

3. Problem: *Body.* I needed help strengthening my physical body so I could stay off caffeine from coffee and have the strength to continue changing *me.*
   Possible Solution: Recognize how much my poor diet was affecting all areas of my life, and that we truly are what we eat and drink.

4. Problem: *Soul.* I needed help in strengthening my soul. I was finally introduced to my soul at the age of 38, when I began drinking tea and making these small changes in my life. Before this, I never once connected to my soul or even thought about it
   Possible Solution: Begin meditating and connecting to the true inner ME.

Right now, I want you to put the book down and go brew a pot of tea and get a pen. Take some time and think about your own life. Fill in the areas of concern below (or in your own journal) and your own possible solutions. Be honest with yourself, especially when it comes to your addictions. We all consistently allow excuses to stop us from us from dieting, exercising, and even taking the time to relax or reflect. It's in this time of reflection that you need to be most honest with yourself. So many of us are addicted to something, whether it is caffeine (like I was), eating, alcohol, drugs, gambling, exercise, sweets, shopping, television, the Internet—you name it. If it's interfering with you getting the most out of life, it's an addiction.

If you can't think of an immediate solution, come back to this page after you finish reading this chapter, or this book, or simply when you're ready. Please don't expect an overnight cure. You've taken 20, 30, 40, 50, or 60 years getting to be the *you* you are. Give yourself a little time to work on becoming the *you* you want to be.

1. Problem: *Addiction.* _____

_____

_____

Possible Solution: _____

_____

_____

_____

_____

_____

2. Problem: *Mind.* _____

_____

_____

Possible Solution: _____

_____

_____

_____

_____

_____

3. Problem: *Body.* _____

_____

_____

Possible Solution: _____

_____

_____

_____

_____

_____

4. Problem: *Soul.* _____

_____

_____

Possible Solution: _____

_____

_____

_____

_____

_____

TEASER

Make It Easier on Yourself: Drink Tea

Don't forget to keep drinking tea during this process. Because of the influence of L-theanine on the brain's alpha waves, changing your reality becomes easier with each cup of tea you drink.

It All Starts with Our Thoughts

Our thoughts are the most powerful tool we own. When we are born we have our own thoughts about what's right for us, but since we cannot speak, we cannot energize them into our reality. So our reality is provided for us by our parents or caregivers.

When we get a little older, we continue to have our own thoughts, but since we live with our parents, they end up controlling our actions; therefore we end up energizing their thoughts and their thoughts become our reality. That's why we revolt the way we do as teenagers! We have our own thoughts about what we want to do, wear, eat, and drink, but we don't have the control to energize them into our realities.

So what do we do?

We sneak off and do as we wish. We begin to energize our own thoughts: I want to drink beer, or I want to go out with this person, or wear that outfit to the party, and these thoughts become our reality. And sometimes the reality we have created, because we are young and inexperienced and foolish, ends up getting us in trouble.

Just when we're on the brink of energizing our own thoughts, we leave home to go to work or to school, to get married, or to live our own lives, and what do we do? We turn over all of our thoughts to our next set of parents, the "hip and cool" group, or the fraternity, sorority, dorm, band, or athletic group at college; our bosses at work; or our significant others. We then energize the thoughts of these groups, making them our reality because we want to be accepted, to fit in, to be loved. We become them! Just like I had become someone other than myself because I wanted to be like everyone else.

Then we see the endless magazines at the checkout counters with pictures and large-type headlines of what the stars are doing, drinking, eating, and wearing. So what do we do? We go right ahead and energize the thoughts of what was right for them, and that becomes our reality (I have to become as thin as Nicole, or as popular as Paris, or as cool as Brad). Or we look at our next-door neighbor who wears a size 2 and lost a ton of weight by taking some pills she got from an infomercial (we don't see that she's also been starving herself). We see someone we envy and think we have to do what they do, be who they are, to be worthwhile ourselves. We don't even realize we're giving away our thoughts.

Own Your Own Thoughts

At the age of 38, I started to take control of my life. Until I realized my life was not mine at all, I thought, "I certainly have enough things around me to validate that I'm in control of my life." I said to myself, "I must be doing something right!" I had been married, I was a successful businessman and sports agent, I lived well, I was part of the "in" crowd, I played polo, I had girlfriends, I traveled the world, I had it going on!

So why was I so miserable? Why didn't I have the strength to handle the tragedies that entered my life? Why was I gaining weight and not working out and not feeling good about myself?

I was allowing myself to energize the thoughts of what others were doing, and making them my reality.

What did I do?

I vowed to make a change. And so can you. You have to say to yourself every day like I did then and still do now, *"I own all of my thoughts, no matter what else is going on in my life or in the lives of others."*

TEASER

Personal Accountability

We are everything we think and say we are.

Everything in life starts out with a thought. Your thoughts, plus the energy you put into them, equals your reality. In order for me to change my reality (which included changing the way I ate and my addiction to caffeine from coffee), I had to change both my thoughts and the focus of my energy.

$I = Sum\ of\ My\ Realities$

$My\ Realities = MY\ Thoughts + Energy$

$Change\ Me = Change\ MY\ Thoughts$

I was going to make a change. So the first thing I did was to create an inventory of the "truths" I believed about myself at the time, trying to be as honest as I possibly could. Of course, there were some positive things. I was a Little League coach in a nearby park, I was donating my time as a high school coach, and eventually I started substitute teaching at Beverly Hills High School. I was a good teacher, and I had a lot to offer.

But at the time, the negatives in my life outweighed the positives. That's why I needed to change. So my inventory fifteen years ago looked like this:

$I = am\ a\ coffee\ drinker$

$I = am\ an\ alcohol\ drinker\ and\ drink\ too\ much\ at\ times$

$I = am\ overweight$

$I = am\ unhappy$

$I = am\ employed$

$I = am\ not\ married$

$I = am\ a\ liar$

$I = am\ not\ working\ out$

$I = am\ not\ eating\ right$

Create an inventory of the things you believe about yourself, being as honest as you can, including some positives as well as negatives.

$I = $ _____

$I = $ _____

I = _____

I = _____

I = _____

I = _____

I = _____

I = _____

I = _____

I = _____

I realized when I made the turn down my new road of life that I had to throw away my old baggage and get a new set. This meant I had to get a grip on everything I was thinking and saying or I would be right back to my coffee pot and my old life.

My life was full of negatives. These were *my* thoughts:

> *I can't drink tea all day.*
> *I can't stop drinking coffee.*
> *I can't eat right.*
> *I can't lose weight.*
> *I can't meditate.*
> *I can't be healthy.*
> *I can't be happy.*
> *I can't stop drinking alcohol.*
> *I can't find love.*
> *I can't work out.*

Make a list of your most prevalent negative thoughts:

_____

_____

_____

_____

_____

_____
_____
_____
_____
_____

Just reading this list can make you depressed. Yet this was how I was living my life. All of these negative "I can't" thoughts, I energized into my realities. I said "I can't" and I couldn't. "I can't" was my excuse for not doing anything, and it's probably yours, too!

I thought I couldn't give up coffee so I didn't.
I thought I couldn't eat right so I stayed heavy.
I thought I couldn't lose weight so I didn't.
I thought I couldn't exercise so I didn't.

That's when I created my simple mantra and wrote it down: *If I say I can, I will. If I say I can't, I won't!*
I wrote my list of positives (I can):

I can drink tea all day.
I can stop drinking coffee.
I can eat right.
I can lose weight.
I can meditate.
I can be healthy.
I can be happy.
I can stop drinking alcohol.
I am a good person.
I can find love.
I can work out.

Reading this list makes you feel strong and ready to take on the world. Within four weeks, I started to feel stronger, more confident, and was finally taking control of ME and my life.

Make a list of positives for yourself:

_____

_____

_____

_____

_____

_____

_____

_____

_____

_____

Don't you feel energized?

When I began by writing down everything I was thinking and energizing to become my reality, I was amazed to see how much of what I was doing all day, I was doing by habit, like drinking coffee instead of asking myself, "Is this what I want to drink? Is this beverage right for me? Do I really like the taste of coffee? Do I like what it's doing to me?" I began to ask myself questions every day:

1. Do I want to drink coffee and get a high from the caffeine?
2. Do I want my heart to pound and my hands to sweat from the caffeine?
3. Do I want to be like everyone else?
4. Do I want that drink of alcohol?
5. Do I want to go out with this woman?
6. Do I want to hang out with this person?
7. Do I want to eat that?
8. Do I want another cup of tea?

9. Do I want to wear this?
10. Do I want to buy that?
11. Do I want to work here and do what I have been doing?
12. Do I want to begin to exercise?

If the answer was yes, I did it, even if it was "bad for me." And that's okay. At least I was taking responsibility for what I was doing. If the answer was no, then I tried my best not to do it. Sometimes I slipped and didn't carry out my intention, but at least I was making progress because I was doing all of this for *me* and not out of the mere habit or because someone else was doing it.

I began to question everything I did and ask myself "Why?"

I began to account for and take responsibility for all of my thoughts. This was where I took the baby steps to taking control of my life.

This is where you will start to take control of your life.

The Business of Life

After I made these lists for myself, I had another epiphany. Unhappy as I was, I was still very successful in my business life. So I asked myself, "What do I do to make my business successful?" The answer? I take my weakest link and make it my strongest. I take an inventory of my business, and then I look not at what I'm doing best, but at what I'm doing worst. And I find the way to turn that weak link around until it becomes the strongest part of my business.

I realized the dichotomy of my personal versus my business life. On the business side, my reality was: "There are no such things as problems, only answers." On the personal side, my reality was: "There are nothing but problems, and there are no answers."

I began to realize that if I wanted to change, I needed to use my business life as a model. I couldn't approach who I was from a negative point of view, constantly thinking there are no answers. I told myself, "You can do this. You can create answers for yourself." I needed solutions. And the first one was to get hold of my thoughts, turn the weakest ones around, and create my new reality.

You can do the same thing. Look at your life as if it was a business. The truth is, most of us are problem solvers. We are problem solvers for our children, for our parents, for our siblings, for our coworkers. Now be one for yourself. You already have the skills you need, you just need to put them into practice.

Bringing It All Back to Tea

With all this talk about "can's" and "can'ts" and weak links, you're probably thinking, "What does tea have to do with all of this?" Tea was the catalyst for all the changes I made in my life. When I was drinking coffee all day, I was "flying" all the time. I was like a souped-up version of the Energizer bunny. My beta brain waves were in a constant state of acceleration, unnecessarily ready for fight or flight. I was so busy *doing* things, I had no time to think about who I was becoming.

It was the tea that calmed me down. Tea evened me out and allowed me to eat right, exercise, lose weight, and make the many changes that led me to the wonderful place I am in today.

You can do it too. Here are a few tricks I learned along the way to make the journey a little bit easier:

* *Find a tea you love to drink.* At this point it doesn't matter where the tea comes from or how much you spend. It just has to be a tea (this does not include Rooibos or herbal tisanes) that you will love to drink all day. I usually recommend to those clients who really love the taste of coffee (very few) our dr. tea's Coffee Tea, which is an oolong tea I have roasted like coffee beans. It looks, smells, and tastes very similar to coffee, but it's a tea. Try lots of different teas and you're bound to find several that really please your palate.

* *Break your "bad" eating habits.* There are many mysteries that science has not yet solved, and bad eating habits is one of them. When we crave certain foods or flavors, part of the problem may be chemical, part may

be mental. But mostly, it's habit, which is a pattern of behavior acquired through frequent repetition. And once the frequent repetition becomes ingrained, it is very difficult to dislodge. Everyone knows that people who smoke cigarettes, for instance, are addicted to nicotine. But what most people don't know is that the addiction to nicotine subsides within a couple of weeks of quitting. It takes much longer to get rid of the *habit* of smoking.

In fact, it is almost impossible to break a habit. Habits fill a vacuum. The only way to get rid of a habit is to replace it with something else, preferably something new and positive in your life. Don't just give up the ice cream, have a Tea Popsicle (page 210) instead. Don't just give up that candy bar; replace it with a cup of tea that tastes like a candy bar. The key is not to focus on what you've stopped doing, but to focus instead on the new behavior that replaces it.

✳ *Break your caffeine addiction.* Do not make the mistake most of us do by going cold turkey on your caffeine/coffee addiction. The act of replacing one cup of coffee with one cup of tea will allow the L-theanine in the tea to slowly cancel out the harmful effects caffeine has put on your system over the years. Here's the plan:

◆ At night, I want you to lay out your tea and tea vessel as you used to lay out your coffee and coffeepot. At work be sure to have a small teapot or strainer and your favorite tea.

◆ The first week, every day, I want you to replace one cup of coffee (or snack or unhealthy food) with at least one cup of your favorite tea.

◆ The second week, every day, I want you to replace two cups of coffee (or snacks or unhealthy foods) with at least two cups of your favorite tea.

◆ The third week, every day, I want you to replace three cups of coffee (or snacks or unhealthy foods) with at least three cups of your favorite tea, and so on.

◆ Drink as much tea during the day as you feel comfortable drinking.

✳ *Realize that it might be tough.* Try to keep drinking your tea all day if you can and if you want to. Don't push it. Listen to your body and what it's saying to you. If you can drink additional cups of your tea during the day then do so, if not, it's okay. If your body is crying out for your iced blended beverage, try to immediately replace the urge with a cup of tea. Better yet, make a Frostea (recipes in chapter 11) drink to quash the urge.

✳ *Use your favorite cup.* This is one of my favorite "tricks": use your favorite coffee cup or vessel while you start this plan. If you're a coffee drinker, chances are, like the rest of us, you always drink it out of the same cup or mug. When you start drinking tea, drink it out of that same cup or mug. If you drink diet soda right out of the can, save your empty cans, rinse them out, and fill them with the tea you love. Then drink your tea right out of the can. Or use a straw—it goes faster. Most people don't have a clue what they're drinking, they like the feel of the can in their hand and it becomes a habit. So pour your tea into the can and drink it that way (you can get plastic covers for open soda cans). If you like to pour your soda into a glass with ice, pour your tea into a glass with ice instead.

✳ *Don't be afraid to drink tea at night.* I thought I could not drink tea at night because of the caffeine. So what I learned was not to drink a fresh cup of tea before going to bed. I instead made my tea and then threw out the liquid of that first pot. Then I added additional water and prepared the next pot and drank from this one. What we have done is called "rinsing," a way to remove just about all of the small amounts of caffeine there is in your first cup or pot of tea because caffeine is very soluble. This is good to do at night, before you sleep, because during sleep your relaxing delta and theta brain waves are doing their jobs and you do not want the beta brain waves stimulated from caffeine to interrupt your precious sleep.

✳ *Realize that it might take time.* Some people have no problem getting over their addiction to caffeine, overeating, or junk food in just a few weeks. But don't be alarmed if it takes you longer. It could take several months (like it did for me), before you will be completely off of your addiction. Just take it slow and steady, stick to it, and say, "I can . . ." I did it and so can you.

There is no trouble so great or grave that cannot be much diminished by a nice cup of tea.

BERNARD-PAUL HEROUX

TEAmmate Profile

Name: Suzy B.
Age: 23
Total Weight Loss: 12
Total Inches Lost: 18.5
Favorite Tea: Strawberry Pie

From the time I was a little kid, all through high school, I was always string-bean skinny. I was really active, and I could eat whatever I wanted to, all day long, without ever having to worry about it. And then I went to college, and started getting older, and discovered beer, and really-bad-for-you food, and everything else. I gained about 25 pounds in four years.

When I graduated from college, I thought that a lot of it would go away since I wouldn't be drinking as much, and I wasn't going to be eating such bad foods—but that didn't happen. And then I went to the doctor for the first time out here and got my blood tested. I found out that, at 23 years old, my cholesterol was already high. That scared the hell out of me. That seems like something you're supposed to worry about when you're much, much older than 23. So I just decided that if I want to be able to live a long, healthy life, that I need to start now.

I was just exhausted all the time. It just felt like I couldn't push myself through the day. Which is not like me at all. I usually have so much energy, and so much life, and I'm just so peppy. But I was not feeling like myself for a long time.

But that all changed when I started the Ultimate Tea Diet. I honestly, absolutely, love drinking the tea. My doctor had also told me I wasn't drinking enough fluids. And then, all of a sudden, we had all these delicious flavors of tea to try and it was so easy to drink the proper amount of fluids throughout the day. And you can use the same leaves several times. So I steep the leaves, and then drink several cups of that kind of tea, and then switch to the next kind, and drink several cups of that kind.

I drink tea from the minute I get into work until the time that I leave. And everybody says, "Oh, there's Suzy with her tea again." I have all my different flavors of tea sitting on my desk, and everybody keeps asking about all of it. Everyone gets excited when I get a new flavor—and now we started trading teas!

But the best part about it, as far as I'm concerned, is when I go home. My roommate's also on the Tea Diet, so we get really excited about cooking food and drinking tea. We have a third roommate, and then we also have a couple of girlfriends who stop over often, and we have a couple of guy friends that live downstairs in our building, and they come up to visit. And every time they come over they say, "Hey, what kind of tea do you have?" So we make pots of tea, and we sit around the table, and it's so social, and calming. We just talk. We don't have to be watching a movie or TV or playing a game, or something else. We're just sitting there, drinking tea, and just enjoying each other.

I've even started exercising again. I go to the gym during the week, and now on the weekends, I've been starting to plan things around activities I want to do. Last weekend, some friends and I went down to the beach, and we Rollerbladed from Santa Monica to Venice—instead of sitting around watching a video.

Now I'm getting compliments about how good I look. A woman at work, whom I hadn't seen in a few months, stopped me in the hallway and said she almost didn't recognize me. And for the first time in years, I can go to the beach and feel comfortable in a bathing suit.

I've been really, really pleased with my results. I didn't have tremendous results for the first couple of weeks. I think it took my body a little bit of time to get used to the changes. The first week, I didn't lose anything; the second week I actually gained two pounds. Then, the third week, I dropped three; and then the fourth week, I dropped another three and I've been losing weight since.

Before I started this, I didn't really believe in dieting, and would rebel against it. This, however, is a diet I really believe in. Because it's all about nutrition, and actually eating right instead of depriving yourself of things your body needs. What I realized, after all these years, is that I wasn't really hungry—I was thirsty! This isn't really a diet, it's educated eating with delicious tea to help you along!

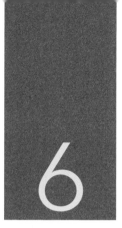

The Process Begins:

Ten Steps to Make Dieting Easier

As I said in the beginning of this book, the object of this book is not just to help you lose weight. It is to help you make changes in your life that will enable you to change your way of eating, and thereby lose weight. My goal is to help you get back the confidence you lost somewhere along the line and to help you gain control of your life. This was evident by the third week of the Ultimate Tea Diet study, as all of the TEAmmates began to feel a certain confidence again in themselves. There was a bounce to their step. They finally had a plan that was easy and made sense so they could incorporate it into their daily lives and it was working just like it did for me and just like it will for you.

Believe me, I know this is not always easy. We're all so good at making excuses: "I'm too busy to stop and make a proper meal." "I'm depressed and I need to eat." "I'm celebrating and I need to eat." "I couldn't find anything healthy on the menu." "It's my birthday." "It's Tuesday." Anything can become an excuse if you let it.

It's your choice. You can let the excuses rule the day, or you can choose—just for this moment—to go another route (just like I went another route fifteen years ago). Just for this moment you can choose a salad over a bowl of pasta, or a turkey burger lettuce wrap (recipe on page 194) over a pastrami on rye. Maybe just for this moment you can choose to forgo the fancy blended high-calorie, high-caffeine beverage you normally drink and make yourself a delicious, healthy cup of tea, a Frostea, or a Hot Todtea (see chapter 11) instead.

We all get tripped up when we try to change everything in our lives all at once. When you say, "I'll never do that again!" don't be surprised if you find yourself falling back on old habits before you know it. Don't try to make a blanket decision that covers the rest of your life—you've done that before and the commitment doesn't last. But you can make one small commitment to yourself right now, and then another small commitment later on, and another and another.

You and I did not put on our extra pounds in one day, one week, or one month. So don't expect to take off all your weight in a day. The tea will help, but it's not magical. You can't expect to put no effort in and still get results. Life doesn't work that way, and neither does losing weight. If you make bigger changes, you'll lose more weight. If you start off slowly, the weight will take more time to come off. But it will come off.

Before you get started, there are a few things you need to do:

1. *Ask yourself this question: Do I really want to lose weight?* This is the most important question you can ask. Ask it now, and if the answer is really, truly "YES," continue reading. If the answer is "NO," put the book away and come on back when you're genuinely ready to lose weight. Because if you really do not want to lose the weight, then nothing you will try will ever work, including the Ultimate Tea Diet, and you will only be fooling yourself and wasting your precious time! You have to really want to make a change in *you;* that's the only way it will work. An easy check to see if you're truly ready is: can you say out loud, *"I can lose weight."* If you can, and do, then you're ready. If you can't, then what you're really saying to yourself is, "I can't lose weight, and I'm really not ready."

As we discussed in the previous chapters about your life and realities, your weight is but another reality of who you are. If you are heavy, no matter what you weigh, it's because you have energized poor eating habits, which have resulted in the reality of being heavier than you desire. But if you're finally ready to make a change, change your reality and you will start to lose weight just like I did and just like every TEAmmate in the Ultimate Tea Diet study.

YOUR LIFE = YOUR thoughts (plan) +
the energy to carry out YOUR thoughts.

Take a close look at these two examples:

Example #1:
Dinner = I'll decide what to eat when I get home from work + I have only enough energy to stick something in the microwave.

Example #2:
Dinner = Tea chicken, vegetables, baked potato, a caramel hot tod-tea for dessert, and tea the rest of the evening (a cup of tea) + the energy I put forth to buy the right foods, plan the meal, and cook them according to the recipes.

You can see for yourself, the person in example #2 really wants to lose weight. She has changed her way of thinking about dinner from "winging it" at the last minute to planning it beforehand. Only then was she able to make the proper meal plan and supply the energy necessary to make it a reality by shopping ahead of time, planning the meal, and preparing the healthy ingredients.

It only works if you truly want to do it. Remember we are changing the way we think about things.

2. *Drink tea all day.* The Ultimate Tea Diet works upon the simple principle of drinking tea all day, every day. It's okay to start slowly. As we said in

the last chapter, if you are currently drinking too much coffee (or diet soda or energy drink or other caffeine-laden beverage), replace one of your usual cups each day with one cup of tea, and drink your tea in your coffee cup until you lose the urge to have coffee. The next week, replace daily two cups of coffee with two cups of tea. Keep going in small increments until you're drinking tea all day. Do the same if you are addicted to sweets like cake or candy, or salty snacks like potato chips or french fries. Find the tea that satisfies that taste (see the next chapter) and replace one snack with a cup of tea. Then replace two snacks, and so on until you find you don't want—or need—the unhealthy snack any longer.

Carry tea with you at all times. Tea bags fit easily in your purse or your pocket. If someone offers you coffee at their home or their office and they don't have tea, you can always ask for hot water, pull out your own bag, and brew away. You can carry a water bottle or thermos of home-brewed tea. You can buy ready-made tea in most delis and grocery stores. Order tea whenever you eat out. It doesn't matter what kind of tea it is. All that matters is that you add tea (white, green, oolong, or black, not Rooibos or herbal blends) all day to your diet plan. The exception is when you are having a trigger or binge food craving, then go to any tea, including a Rooibos or herbal blend, instead of eating your binge food.

We know from hundreds of scientific studies (some of which you learned about in chapter 3) that drinking tea actually suppresses appetite and helps to keep excess body fat under control. One particular study that appeared in the 2005 *Annals of Nutrition & Metabolism* showed that supplementation with EGCG abolishes—actually stops—diet-induced obesity (that means they purposely fed the test subjects a high-fat diet in order to get them to gain weight). The study concluded, "Dietary supplementation with EGCG should be considered as a valuable natural treatment option for obesity."

When you drink tea all day, your body is working to metabolize the tea into your blood system through your stomach. When the L-theanine from the tea hits your brain, it acts as a mood and appetite stabilizer, giving you that satisfied feeling you have after you've just finished eating. As the day goes on and you continue to consume your tea, it continues to stimulate your body's thermogenesis (fat burning processes).

The next time you have the urge to eat, especially when you're not physically hungry, drink some tea instead. Two things will happen: first, the urge to eat will diminish, and then, when your body tells you it's time to eat a meal, you'll find that you are eating less.

3. *Identify the foods that trigger you to binge or overeat.* Remember the commercial that used to say, "Bet you can't eat just one?" That ad referred to potato chips, and it was so true. It's almost impossible to eat just one chip. Some people are able to eat just a handful, and then walk away. For others, nothing less than the entire bag will do. If you're one of those people, then potato chips are a trigger food for you.

Trigger foods trigger binges. They're the foods we'll go out to get in a blinding snowstorm or at midnight when there's already plenty of food in the house. They tend to be high in sugar or fat or both. They have little to do with being hungry (although if you're very hungry, trigger foods are usually much harder to resist). If you feel that you're out of control around a particular food, you've got to eliminate it from your reality. If you love to eat ice cream, for instance, and cannot stop at one or two scoops but must finish the half-gallon, then you *cannot* have ice cream in your house. You *cannot order ice cream* for dessert when you are out and about. This goes for anything you are compulsive over: candy, doughnuts, fries, beer, cakes, potatoes, gum, cookies, breads, or anything that triggers you to eat more than you want to. If you really want to lose the weight and change your reality, then:

> *Stop buying these foods for home.*
> *Stop ordering them when out.*
> *Stop eating your trigger foods.*

Find a tea, Rooibos, or herbal blend you love instead and drink that tea whenever you have the urge to have your trigger food. This really does work and in chapter 7 we have provided you with a list of teas, Rooibos, and herbal blends identified from our Ultimate Tea Diet study to satisfy the desire to eat some of the most common binge foods.

4. *Plan your meals.* Remember, everything you do starts with your thoughts. Begin your day by thinking about eating healthy foods and meals from breakfast through dinner. Think about what you plan to have, then write it down. Put your energy into executing the plan by eating what you've set forth in your plan. Make it fun, not a chore. Make sure you "mix it up"; nothing sabotages a diet like eating the same boring meal over and over again. The Ultimate Tea Diet gives you an incredible array of choices and recipes, many of which are made with tea.

5. *Eat only when you are hungry and stop when you're full.* This sounds like plain old common sense, but I know how difficult it is to do. Habits are hard to break, and the habit of eating to fill emotional needs is one of the most difficult. But aren't you tired of being tired because nothing has worked for you before? Then it's time to listen to your body and eat when it tells you it needs to refuel. Don't eat because you're having a bad day, or because you're having a good day, or because someone else you're with is hungry. Stop eating when you're full—or better yet, before you're full, since it takes about twenty minutes for the brain to signal the body that it's had enough to eat. It's not a crime to leave food on your plate, despite what your mother may have told you. You can jazz up leftovers by adding tea to them when you reheat them, or by using a condiment (like ketchup, mustard, or mayo) spiced with tea.

6. *Do not eat between meals.* Drink tea instead. I tell you that because it's what I do, and it's what has worked for me. Of course, I want you to consult your doctor or health professional before you go on this or any other diet. If you have problems with blood sugar, he or she may suggest that you eat something every three or four hours. If that's the case, have one of the healthy snacks included in the Ultimate Tea Diet Meal

Plan, or choose one from the list starting on page 148. Otherwise, eat only your planned meals and drink as much tea as you like in between. When you want to reach for a snack, have a cup of tea first, wait fifteen to twenty minutes, and then see if you still feel the need for something to eat. If you do, and because this plan is all about you, make it a smart choice. If you are eating balanced Tea Diet meals in conjunction with drinking your favorite tea throughout the day, your cravings and need to eat when you're not hungry will go away. This usually happens within a few days to a week of implementing the Ultimate Tea Diet.

7. *Breakfast is a* must. Plan on having something for breakfast within one hour of rising each and every day for the rest of your life, even if it's just a piece of fruit. In this case, your mother was right—breakfast is the most important meal of the day. A healthy, balanced breakfast (with a cup of tea, of course) is the fuel that enables you to have a strong start on your day's adventures.

8. *Replace bad eating habits with a cup of tea.* We all have certain habits we developed when we were young and have kept up most of our lives. I had to have a candy bar before bed each and every night. If I couldn't get my candy bar, I had ice cream with cake. When I started on my own Ultimate Tea Diet, I didn't have all of the teas and tisanes that are available today in the stores and on line. So I made my own replacement tea by adding bits of chocolate and caramel to my teapot. I replaced my late-night sweet tooth (approximately 500 calories) with a cup of my own sweet tea (5 calories). I drank my candy bar replacement tea until I satisfied my sweet tooth and then went to bed. I was able to fall asleep immediately because I didn't go to bed high on a sugar rush. I awoke feeling great—no sugar hangover—and confident in knowing I was on the right track and full of energy. In chapter 7 you'll find a handy list of tea flavors and in chapter 11 you'll find recipes to make your own replacement tea that will help satisfy a variety of cravings.

Follow this simple but most important rule: If what you are about to eat is not on your plan for the day, or you have the urge to have a candy bar, potato chips, coffee, or whatever is your particular bad habit, find a suitable tea to replace your desire or habit like I did, and watch the pounds disappear while you add pure natural good health to your body.

TEASER

Breaking the Late-Night Habit

Many people who come into dr. tea's tell me their habit is not so much a particular food as it is eating late at night. It becomes a habit that's difficult to break. If you feel you must have something late at night, don't go for a trigger food. First go for tea. Then, if you must, choose a healthy snack. Have a low-fat yogurt with some loose tea mixed in, or a piece of fruit with your favorite sweet tea. The tea will help you reduce the nighttime eating impulse over a period of time.

Will it be difficult to get over the hump? Every addiction is tough to break. The tea might not satisfy you in the beginning, but soon the L-theanine will begin to work on the dopamine and serotonin to calm those urges and help you break the late-night habit.

I didn't successfully go cold turkey from sweets; I still had nights where I had to have my candy bar. But these evening cravings slowly gave way, and I looked forward to having my tea instead.

9. *Enjoy being a tea drinker.* Ignore the old stereotypes that tell you tea is for the "pinkies up" crowd, or for little old ladies, or for pairing with crumpets or cucumber sandwiches. The truth is that tea is hip, tea is healthy—and tea is sexy. Let me explain. I used to think that I had to order coffee to be macho and to do what everyone else did. But when I started to change my life and began drinking tea, a funny thing

happened. I would go out to dinner with a date and order tea when the meal was over. And women began to look at me in a different light. They said I was sensitive. They said I listened. I thought they were kidding me; after all, hadn't I always listened? No, I hadn't. I'd been so wired on coffee, all I could hear were my own thoughts racing around my brain. When the tea started affecting my alpha brain waves, I really did become a better listener! And suddenly I was more popular than ever with the ladies. Who knew what a simple cup of tea could do! And it's not just men who become sexier. It's not sexy to be jumpy and anxious and tense from caffeine or from too much sugar and junk food. It is sexy when your skin is clear, your eyes are bright, your hair is shiny, you're calm and centered, your clothes fit well, and you are the most confident woman in the room. (Makes you want to have another cup of tea right now, doesn't it?)

10. *Don't expect perfection.* We are all human. We all mess up. I did and you will, too. When you do, move on. Go right back to your tea. Learn from your mistake; it just might be the reminder you need of how you felt before you began the Ultimate Tea Diet. I remember "sneaking" a candy bar one night early on. I woke up at 4:00 a.m. and couldn't get back to sleep. When I finally did, I slept fitfully and woke up wanting a cup of coffee. I had no appetite. I felt so poorly that it actually helped me make a better choice the next time I had the urge for a sweet treat at night. Do not get bogged down in what you did—get energized about what you will do from now on.

You might find one day you have a jones for your favorite caffeinated drink. This happened to me when I was trying to give it up. One night I got lazy and forgot to pick up some tea after I ran out. The next morning I went to the shopping center in Malibu to get some. I pulled into a parking space, looked up, and there it was: the ubiquitous coffee shop. I was helpless. I could smell the aroma of the coffee putting me into a trance. Before I knew it, I found myself sitting down and having my old drug of choice: a regular coffee with a shot of espresso. And you know something, it was great! I felt right at home. And for a few minutes, I felt wonderful. Then in about twenty minutes I started to feel that old feeling. My heart began racing and I was ready for action. I had lost my grounded, centered state and instead there I was, all over the place. I had to get out of there. I went to the parking lot and couldn't even find my car.

So I went back into the coffee shop and ordered a cup of tea. I drank it down and waited until the L-theanine kicked in and leveled me off. You too may forget to have your tea one day, or run out and forget to buy more. You too may decide to have just one cup of coffee, or a candy bar, or a bag of chips. It's okay. It's not the end of the world. Here's what you need to remember: It's not that we've messed up that counts; it's how long it takes us to get back on track. So if you should find yourself in a state of human imperfection, don't be so hard on yourself. Go right back to your tea and the easy steps above. Brew your tea and drink it often. Go back to your plan and get back on track just like the TEAmmates of our Ultimate Tea Diet study group did.

This is why the Ultimate Tea Diet works: because we finally have something easy to go back to when we mess up—tea. Tea is easy. Tea is everywhere. And tea will become your best friend, as it has become mine. So go ahead and get yourself another cup and let's get to the diet.

If man has no tea in him, he is incapable of understanding truth and beauty.

JAPANESE PROVERB

TEAmmate Profile

Name: Bill B.

Age: 26

Total Weight Loss: 31

Total Inches Lost: 26.5

Favorite Tea: Orange Matcha Powder

I have dieted several times before. I usually start it, and then realize that it's too diffi-cult to do, and I just give up on it. But this is a lot easier than most other diets I've found. At first I didn't believe it would work. I thought, "I'll definitely always have the cravings." But once I started replacing them with tea it seemed to help me actually not feel like I really, really need to eat cheeseburgers all the time.

Or I can actually tell myself: No, you don't need to get into that fridge. You don't need to eat that. You're not actually hungry. I am able to think more clearly, and I find more activities to fill up the time I usually spent preparing or eating food. I've changed what I had normally been eating. I used to be a steak-and-sausage type of guy. And now I'm more of a chicken-and-turkey type of dude. I've actually tried using tea as marinades, and it really tastes great.

And, since I'm putting more exercise into my repertoire, I've been finding that I've been having a lot more fun with my life. I've been going to a lot of different hik-ing trails in national parks, which is just wonderful for my cardio. I fill up water bot-tles with iced tea, instead of water, and off I go!

I'm not sure exactly how much weight I've lost, but I've dropped belt sizes up the wazoo. One morning I went to buckle my belt and pulled it closed and realized there was no hole to put the buckle in. I had run out of holes; I needed a whole new belt. I didn't just go down a couple notches—I needed a whole new, smaller belt.

Then I went to my old roommate's birthday party and saw a bunch of people I haven't seen in a couple of months. They were not only amazed at my awesome weight loss, they also said I look much younger. My roommate, who has seen me fairly often over the last four years, said, "Wow, dude. I'm not kidding. You look like you did in your high school picture!" Now he's started drinking tea, too.

7

Find the Tea You Love

Everyone who comes to dr. tea's or sees me on television or hears me on the radio talking about the Ultimate Tea Diet asks the same question: "How do I get started?" And I give everyone the same answer: "Find a tea you love and drink it all day."

Of course, that doesn't mean you need to find just one tea and stick to it, forgoing all others. That would deprive you of the many wonders of the world of tea! I urge everyone to try many different teas, hot or cold, until they find the *ones* they love the best. If you eat the same foods over and over again, you're bound to get bored, and the same goes for tea.

So this chapter is going to be a reference guide to tea and how to find which teas suit you best. There are light teas, sweet teas, spicy teas, heavy teas, teas that taste like licorice, teas that have a fruity taste, teas that taste like pumpkin pie. There are teas that remind you of your grandmother's hugs, teas that fill your senses with a hint of springtime, and teas with smoky flavors that bring back memories of wintry days in front of a fireplace. There are teas that you will choose to drink all day, and there are teas that you may choose to satisfy a particular yen, like the cravings teas you will find later on.

I can't tell you which teas you are going to love, and I would never tell you which teas to drink. This book is all about you; you are an individual with your own preferences, your own personality, and you will have your own favorites. Once again, let your taste buds be your guide.

I do understand, however, that if you are just beginning your journey to becoming a tea drinker, you may find all the choices intimidating. After all, there are the four basic kinds of tea (white, green, oolong, and black), and then there are all the flavor choices within each type (that is, there are many different kinds of black tea, green tea, etc., not to mention all the teas blended with various flavors). So how do you decide?

I could give you some technical advice on tasting tea the way experts do it. They taste tea the same way wine tasters taste wine—they swish it around and spit it out (mostly because they have more tea to taste and do not want to get full by drinking a whole cup of each tea). Tea tasters, like wine tasters, have an extensive vocabulary to describe what they're tasting, including:

* Body: the "weight" of the tea on the tongue (light, medium, or heavy)
* Bouquet: the aroma that enters the nose when sniffing the tea
* Bright: tea that is fresh and of high quality
* Brisk: pungent without being too high in tannin
* Flat: used to describe a tea that is old or stale
* Flavor: the sensation perceived on the tongue as sweet, salty, sour, or bitter
* Full-bodied: an ideal combination of color and flavor
* Long in the mouth: describes a tea that leaves a long-lasting impression in the front and back of the mouth
* Refined: describes teas that are both delicate and subtle

The more tea you taste, the better you'll become at discerning all the qualities listed above. But the truth is, you don't need any of those descriptive phrases. All you really need is to answer the question, "Do I like this tea?" And basically, the best way to answer that question is to try as many different varieties from as many different manufacturers and tea purveyors as possible, and stock up on the ones that suit you best.

What Does Tea Taste Like?

The comedian David Steinberg tells a joke I have always loved: "Trying to describe my life to my parents," he said, "is like trying to describe a cranberry to a Martian." This joke always comes to mind when people ask me what the four basic tea types taste like. It's almost impossible to answer, because there are so many varieties of each, but here are some basic concepts:

* *White tea* is often described as light and slightly sweet. It is pale in color, and does not have as strong an aroma as green or black tea.

* *Green tea* sometimes has a bit of a "grassy" taste, and some people find it slightly bitter. The degrees of flavor differ quite a bit from one green tea to another, as there are so many varieties.

* *Oolong tea* has a well-balanced taste and aroma, but it also has a wide range—from teas that are close to green to teas that are nearly black. Oolong is often brewed to be strong, and typically leaves a sweet aftertaste.

* *Black tea* is the most astringent of the teas, meaning that it has a higher tannin content. Some people enjoy black tea best by adding milk or lemon juice; others like their black tea "black."

These are bases to which all ingredients are added to make flavored teas. However, because each type of tea has so many varieties, you may want to try several "pure" (unflavored) teas first and then move on to those with other flavors added.

The Flavors of Tea

If you can think of a flavor you love, you can probably find it in a tea. And you can probably find several versions of it. For instance, if you like orange, you are just as likely to find a green tea with orange flavor added as you are a black-tea-and-orange combination. Any type of tea can be made into a flavored tea—in fact, flavoring technology has improved so much in recent years that tea purveyors are limited mostly by their imaginations (and their taste buds) in designing new flavors for their customers. Here is just a partial list of the flavors of tea you can now find in your local supermarket and/or tea salons:

Almond	*Cream*	*Peach*
Apple	*Currant*	*Pineapple*
Apricot	*Ginger*	*Plum*
Banana	*Grapefruit*	*Pomegranate*
Blackberry	*Jasmine*	*Raspberry*
Blueberry	*Lemon*	*Rum*
Caramel	*Licorice*	*Spice*
Cherry	*Lime*	*Strawberry*
Chocolate	*Lychee*	*Tiramisu*
Cinnamon	*Mango*	*Toffee*
Coconut	*Melon*	*Vanilla*
Coffee	*Orange*	

There are also some fairly well-known varieties of tea that you have probably come across in your local supermarket, tea salon, or restaurant—some of which have been popular in the western world for several hundred years, and others that are just now becoming "rising stars" in the rapidly expanding universe of teas in both bags and loose leaf formats. Here is a brief sampling:

✴ *Assam:* This tea is named after the region in northeastern India in which it is grown. Discovered to be growing in this region after the Opium Wars between China and England, it is the second largest tea production region in the world, after China, and produces more than 1,500,000 pounds of tea annually. It is a full-bodied tea with a strong, bright color and a brisk, malty flavor.

✴ *Chai:* What has recently become a very popular drink in coffee and tea shops in this country has been served for hundreds of years in India and

South Asia. In fact, the word "chai" actually means tea, so when you ask for a chai tea, you are asking for a tea tea. It is properly called *masala chai*, and is sold by street vendors called "chai wallahs" on trains, in bus stations, and on the street in most Indian neighborhoods. It is traditionally prepared by boiling loose leaf black tea in a pot with milk and water and added spices including cardamom, cinnamon, ginger, cloves, and pepper (although the specific spices vary from region to region). In some regions, they also add honey. They then place a sugar cube in the bottom of the teacup and pour the chai over it. Chai is more popular in India than coffee.

* *Darjeeling:* This is another Indian tea that comes from the Darjeeling province in the foothills of the Himalayas. It is known as the Champagne of black teas, and is considered one of India's finest teas. There are two categories of Darjeeling tea, depending on when the leaves are harvested. What is known as "first flush"—considered to be the finest and most expensive—is harvested from late February to the middle of April, and produces a light-green tea with a brisk, pleasant flavor. The "second flush" is harvested in June; these teas are fuller-bodied with an amber color and a slightly fruity taste.

* *Earl Grey:* This tea was named after a real person, Charles Grey, the second Earl Grey, who was British Prime Minister from 1830 to 1834. There are many different stories of how Earl Grey's name was placed on the tea. One is that he was given the recipe by a Chinese mandarin whose life he had saved. Another version of the story says that he was given the tea after one of his servants rescued the son of an Indian raja from a tiger. Another is that the teas from India at the time were very young, as was the tea industry in that country. The teas did not have the richness of the Chinese teas to which the English had become accustomed, so Earl Grey ordered the addition of oil of bergamot, a small acidic orange, to his tea to take away the bitter taste, and the rest, as they say, is history.

* *English Breakfast:* This is a full-bodied blend of several types of black tea with light floral undertones. It has been said that when it is mixed with

milk, it produces an aroma that is reminiscent of warm toast and honey. The surprising fact is that English Breakfast tea was actually invented in Edinburgh, Scotland by a tea merchant named Drysdale who simply called it "Breakfast Tea." There is also a similar tea that we know as Irish Breakfast tea, but in Ireland it is simply known as "tea."

＊ *Gunpowder:* One of the first teas to be exported from China to the West, this green tea, originally from the Guangdong province of China, got its name because it is made up of leaves hand-rolled into tiny pellets which explode to many times their size in hot water (today, most gunpowder tea is rolled by machines). It is a full-bodied tea with a hint of smokiness. Some tea drinkers say it also has a slightly peppery taste. In the cup, it has a yellow color. It can also be mixed with peppermint or any other herb or flavor you enjoy.

＊ *Matcha:* This Japanese green tea is different from most other teas in that it is a powder that you put into a cup or bowl, add hot water to, stir until frothy, and drink. Unlike most other teas, the leaves themselves (in their powdered form) are consumed. This is the strongest of the green teas, has a thicker consistency than most teas, and has a bittersweet taste. It is also used to make green tea ice cream and some Japanese candies. Matcha is the tea that is used in the traditional Japanese tea ceremony.

＊ *Orange Pekoe:* There is no orange flavor in orange pekoe. This term doesn't even refer to a distinctive type of tea; it is, instead, a term used to refer to a grade of tea consisting of large pieces of leaves or even whole leaves. In order to be graded as orange pekoe, the tea must be obtained from new flushes and consist of the leaf bud and several of the youngest leaves.

The word pekoe may have come from a corrupted version of *Bai Hoa,* the Chinese word for white tip, referring to the white down that covers the leaf bud. The tea was originally brought from China to Holland, where it was presented to the royal family, the House of Orange. Thenceforth, it became known as orange pekoe.

✳ *Sencha:* Sencha means green (sen) tea (cha) in Japanese. This green tea is the most popular type of tea in Japan today. Sencha is light green in color, and is both sweet and bitter at the same time. It is sometimes mixed with popped and roasted rice, and referred to as *genmaicha.*

The Tea Quiz

Now that you have familiarized yourself with some of the teas available to you, you still may be asking, "Where do I start?" (If you already are drinking your favorite teas then skip this section and continue drinking what you love until you want to try something new.)

My first answer is always going to be: "Try as many kinds of tea as you can, and find the ones you love!" However, I realize that some of you would like some help in narrowing your options. So take the mini quiz below and find out what type of tea just might suit you best.

1. What is your favorite ice cream flavor?
    A. Vanilla
    B. Mint chocolate chip
    C. Banana split with chocolate syrup, nuts, and cherries

2. What is your favorite dining experience?
    A. Four-star restaurant
    B. Fast-food restaurant
    C. Backyard barbeque

3. What is your favorite type of food?
    A. Light salad and broiled salmon
    B. Burgers and dogs
    C. Spicy ethnic dishes

4. You have an unexpected day off from work. Would you be more likely to:
    A. Visit a museum
    B. Spend the day at the beach
    C. Ride the roller coaster at an amusement park

5. Which beverage do you prefer to drink (besides tea, of course)?
   A. Wine
   B. Beer
   C. Coffee

6. Which of these movie stars would be your ideal mate (ignoring their gender)?
   A. Helen Mirren
   B. Chris Rock
   C. Bruce Willis

Now, before you tally your score, realize that in tea drinking, as in life, nothing is purely black and white—or in this case, white, green, oolong, or black. Every black tea drinker has a bit of white tea in them as well, and vice versa. But if you are looking for a place to get started, here are some hints according to your quiz results:

If most of your answers fell into the *A* category, you will probably enjoy a more sophisticated, refined tea, such as:

Jasmine Pearl Green Tea
White Teas
Pu-Erh Teas

If most of your answers fell into the *B* category, you will probably enjoy a tea that's a bit heartier, such as:

Earl Grey
Black Teas in general
Roasted Oolong Teas

If most of your answers fell into the *C* category, you will probably enjoy a spicier, fun, more full-bodied tea, such as:

Lapsang Souchong
Spicy Chai Black Teas
Fruit-flavored Teas

And remember, there are no judgments here. One tea is not better or better for you than any other. It's simply a matter of taste. And just because this quiz has pegged you as a Jasmine Pearl drinker doesn't mean you might not also enjoy a Darjeeling or a spicy Chai.

In fact, here are some other criteria you might find useful:

✳ What is your favorite flavor?

If you answered mint, for instance, there are many varieties of mint tea you might like. If you're a fan of blueberries, look for a tea that will satisfy those berry-loving taste buds. Try several and find the ones that make you feel the best.

TEASER

Keep True Tea in Mind

Remember that if you are drinking tea for the purposes of losing weight, you should be drinking true tea that comes from the *Camellia sinensis* plant. If you choose an herbal or Rooibos tisane, you may like the taste, but you won't get the Tea3 benefits. What you can do is simply add a small amount of white, green, oolong, or black tea to your beloved herbal or Rooibos tisane from a bag or in loose leaf form and you have just added the Tea3 benefits to your favorite taste, and created a tea from a tisane.

✳ Are you a purist? Do you like your coffee black and your food free of condiments? Do you prefer your clothes with classic lines and your accessories chic and smart? You will probably appreciate your tea straightforward—a "plain" white, green, oolong, or black will do, without additional flavors.

✳ Do you prefer to mix things up? If you're more likely to add a little bling to your wardrobe, go out for a spicy meal, and have a spirit of adventure, the sky is the limit as far as your tea choices are concerned. You might like a Masala Chai, a complex Darjeeling, or a tea that combines exotic flavors such as dr. tea's French Lemon Ginger Sherbet.

Have a Craving? Have Some Tea

On the Ultimate Tea Diet, there are actually two reasons for drinking tea. We've discussed the first throughout the book so far: so that the weight-loss properties of the caffeine, L-theanine, and EGCG can enhance thermogenesis, work on your body's alpha waves, and help you burn more energy and curb your appetite. Now we come to the second reason for drinking tea: to satisfy a particular craving so that you are less likely to binge on a trigger food.

If you remember my story from chapter 6, you will remember my obsession with having a candy bar each night before going to sleep. The obsession was like a force inside me I couldn't resist. I wanted that taste of chocolate and caramel. I don't know if it was a physiological need I was trying to satisfy or a psychological one; all I know is I had what the dictionary defines as a craving—an intense desire for some particular thing. My particular thing was that candy bar.

You may find that simply by drinking tea all day—any tea—your cravings naturally diminish. That is probably due to L-theanine's calming effect and its influence on your alpha brain waves. But if that doesn't do the trick for you, you may want to find a tea you drink for the express purpose of satisfying the hankering you have for what would normally be a trigger food.

So here comes the exception to one of my basic rules—the one that says you should be drinking true teas that come from my favorite Cami plant. If you find a true tea that satisfies your flavor craving, all the better. But if you don't—if your "craving" tea is Rooibos-based or is an herbal blend tisane, that is okay. This is not the tea you will be drinking all day; this is a tisane you will save for those times when you're longing for a food that is not on your plan. Remember if your craving is late at night, like mine was, prepare the tea, throw out the first steep and drink from the second and subsequent caffeine-free steeps; you won't have to do that with tisanes, as they are caffeine-free.

Many customers come into dr. tea's and ask me to recommend teas for them. I tell them to drink whichever tea they love. If they want to lose weight, I tell them about the Ultimate Tea Diet. More often than not, at the end of our conversation, the customer will say, "There's just one thing, Dr. Tea. I'm a chocoholic," or "I love to have a piece of cherry pie for dessert," or "I don't know if I can give up my ice cream treat every night."

"Ah," I say, "I have just the thing for you!" And in my most "doctorly" voice I add, "Take one cup or as many pots as you need of this tea or tisane the next time you have a craving, and call me in the morning." I love to get their phone calls or e-mails a few days later or speak to them again when they come back to dr. tea's. They all tell me about how they are able, with the help of their craving tea or tisane, to finally give up what had become a problem food for them, just like my candy bar cravings became a thing of the past for me.

Identify Your Craving

The first thing you have to do is identify your craving, the same way you identified your trigger food(s). These may be one and the same, or they may be different (you may crave chocolate, but pizza is your trigger food). Your cravings may change as well. One night you may crave something sweet; other times you may want something salty. But as with trigger foods, most people have their favorites that they crave most often. If you keep a variety of teas on hand, you will always have choices that meet your desires.

If you often crave a candy bar at night, as I did, take a look at the key ingredients. If the candy bar has chocolate and caramel in it, find a tea that has chocolate or caramel or both as added flavors. If it has coconut, look for a coconut tea. Come fall, if you find yourself lusting for a piece of pumpkin pie, find a pumpkin-flavored tea (or try Chai, which has similar spices to those usually used in making pumpkin pie). If you're ordering over the Internet and can't taste or smell the tea before you try it, buy a small quantity at first to be sure the tea tastes like the item you're craving.

The list of teas below is just to give you an idea of the kinds of flavored teas you can use to titillate your taste buds in place of some high-calorie confections you are currently consuming. You don't have to use dr. tea's teas. You can find flavored loose leaf or bagged teas in the supermarket from many different manufacturers. You may have a tea shop in your neighborhood with similar blends. Or you can go on the Internet, search for "chocolate tea" (or whatever your craving flavor might be) and come up with any number of places where you can order tea online.

Ultimate Tea Diet Craving Teas from dr. tea's

CANDY:

1. Dr. Tea's Candy Bar Black Tea
2. Licorice Oolong Tea
3. Caramel Rooibos (tisane)
4. Mint Chocolate Chip Ice Cream Rooibos (tisane)

CHOCOLATE:

1. Dr. Tea's Candy Bar Black Tea
2. Chocolate Hazelnut Torte Rooibos (tisane)
3. Tiramisu Rooibos (tisane)
4. Mint Chocolate Chip Ice Cream Rooibos (tisane)
5. Chocolate Bliss Cake (tisane)
6. Chocolate and Roses Rooibos (tisane)

VANILLA:

1. Vanilla Berry Truffle (tisane)
2. Vanilla Rooibos (tisane)

3. Hojicha de la Crème Green Tea

4. Earl Grey a la Crème Black Tea

ICE CREAM AND SHERBETS

1. Mint Chocolate Chip Ice Cream Rooibos (tisane)

2. Passion Fruit Rooibos (tisane)

3. Orange Sherbet Green Tea

4. Pineapple Green Tea

5. Dr. Tea's Candy Bar Black Tea

6. Mango Green Tea

7. French Lemon Ginger (tisane)

8. Dr. Tea's Own Coffee Oolong Tea

9. Black Lichee Tea

10. Key Lime Pie (tisane)

11. Caramel Rooibos (tisane)

12. Jasmine Green Tea

13. Moroccan Mint Green Tea

14. Plum Oolong Tea

15. Lichee and Cantaloupe White Tea

PIES, CAKES AND COOKIES

1. Blueberry White Pie Tea

2. Peach Pie White Tea

3. Pineapple Coconut Pie White Tea

4. Strawberry Pie Green Tea

5. Pineapple Green Tea

6. Black Apple Pie Tea

7. Apple Pie Rooibos (tisane)

8. Chocolate Hazelnut Torte Rooibos (tisane)

9. Tiramisu Rooibos (tisane)

10. Peach Pie Green Tea

11. Ginger Bread Rooibos (tisane)

12. Strawberry Raspberry Herbal Dream Rooibos (tisane)

13. Orange Pound Cake Rooibos
14. Orange Spice Cake Rooibos (tisane)
15. Chocolate Bliss Cake (tisane)
16. Cinnamon Roll (tisane)
17. Mango Green Tea
18. Key Lime Pie Rooibos (tisane)
19. Caramel Rooibos (tisane)
20. Chocolate Cream Pie
21. Cherry Pie Green Tea
22. Orange Spice Cake Black Tea
23. Pumpkin Pie Rooibos (tisane)
24. Yoga Herbal Chai (tisane)

FRENCH FRIES AND POTATO CHIPS:

You can drink the tea, eat the tea, or break up the leaves and add them to your food.

1. Tai Ping Green Tea
2. Sencha Green Tea (add salt)

POPCORN:

1. Genmaicha Green Tea

BAR B QUE:

1. Lapsang Souchong Black Tea

You will notice that several of the teas on this list are Rooibos-based tisanes. To my knowledge, there have been no studies done that prove Rooibos to have weight-loss properties (although it has a high number of antioxidants, so it's a very healthy drink). But as we have mentioned before, all you have to do is add a small amount of white, green, oolong, or black tea to the Rooibos tisane and you have yourself a true tea. And some of these teas, because of the added ingredients, may have 5 or 6 calories per 8-ounce cup. But to my way of thinking, if you're drinking a 5-calorie cup of tea versus a 500-calorie gooey dessert, you've just eliminated 495 unnecessary calories and added all of the health and weight-loss benefits of tea.

TEASER

A Tip of Last Resort

If you have put in a good faith effort and still can't find a tea to satisfy your craving, try making one yourself. That is what I did before I became a tea purveyor, as I explained earlier. I used my favorite candy bar. You can use your favorite craving flavor. If licorice is the flavor you crave, cut off a small piece of a licorice stick or take one piece of Good & Plenty and mix it into a cup of tea.

The problem is, of course, that in order to do that, you have to have your craving food in the house, which I do not recommend. Once you have cut off a piece of a chocolate bar, it may be too much of a temptation or struggle to put the rest away for your next cup of tea. Many times I found myself taking a bite of the candy bar or, even worse, eating the whole thing while my tea was steeping. But I had no other choice at the time. If that's the case, my advice is "Don't try this at home." Go back and try another search for a tea that will do the trick, or e-mail me drtea@ultimateteadiet.com and we can discuss it.

Or rather than adding an actual piece of candy to your tea, you can try adding your own flavorings. For instance, you can use vanilla beans, coffee beans, cinnamon sticks, or sugar-free extracts like vanilla, almond, rum, caramel, chocolate, or butter pecan. Be sure to read the labels before you use these extracts so you're sure they are sugar-free. At dr. tea's we use stevia, a natural sweetener from a plant that comes in many flavors with zero to a few calories. Be adventurous. You just might come up with something delicious!

A Tea for All Seasons

One of the best things about tea is that you can enjoy the same kind of tea year-round, or you can change the type of tea you drink to fit the season (or the occasion or your mood or any other criteria). But there are some teas that go particularly well with changes in the weather and that mirror the type of seasonal foods you may eating.

In the spring, when a tea drinker's fancy turns to love and rejuvenation, try a Mint Tea, a Chamomile, a Jasmine Pearl, a Blueberry White Tea, or a tea infused with rosebuds.

In the summer, we usually eat a lighter fare than we do at other times of the year. In most parts of the country, it's a time to enjoy fresh, delicious fruits. So it seems like a perfect time to try some of the teas blended with fruit flavors like pineapple, blueberry, coconut, strawberry, passion fruit, raspberry, lemon, lime, and peach—or by adding two tablespoons of fresh fruit right into your teapot.

In the fall, when you start to notice a chill in the air, you want something a little warmer, something that will fill up your senses and get you ready for the long winter months ahead. There's something about cinnamon that shouts out cardigans and falling leaves. This is the time you might want to try a Pumpkin Tea, a Ginger Bread, a Caramel, a Chai, a Black Orange Spice variety, or you might want to try adding a dash of cinnamon to your tea.

And then it's winter. It's cold out. You're spending more time indoors. You want a "serious" tea, perhaps a straightforward black tea, an Earl Grey, or even a Pu Erh. And for the holidays, how about an Egg Nog or Rum Raisin Black Tea?

More than anything, it's simply what you like. If you like a "summery" white tea with blueberry in the middle of winter, that's what you should be drinking. There are no rules here, only what makes you feel good.

Tea to Go

If I asked you to drink coffee all day every day (which I would never do), it wouldn't be a difficult task, as coffee is available everywhere. With tea—not as much. However, thanks to the fact that more and more people are discovering the tastes of tea every day—and its amazing health benefits—that is rapidly changing. It is now easier than ever before for you to be drinking tea all day, every day.

Obviously, I don't expect you to be at home every day brewing pot after pot. But I do hope that you will take tea with you wherever you go or have it available wherever you are. This is not at all difficult, but it may take a bit of planning until it becomes part of your lifestyle. Here are some suggestions:

* *Develop a morning ritual.* If you used to be a coffee drinker, you probably had a ritual associated with making your coffee. Many people I know grind their own beans, set them up in the coffee maker before they go to bed, set the timer, and have their coffee waiting for them in the morning. They then pour coffee into their travel cups and enjoy the brew in the car or train as they travel to work. You can do almost the same thing with tea. You can rinse your vessel with hot water, then coat the bottom with tea, ready for your morning brew. You can use a coffee maker with a timer to have hot water waiting for you in the pot when you get up, then follow the steeping instructions you learned in chapter 2. Let it steep for two to three minutes, pour it into your travel cup, and you're off for the day!

* *Prepare bottles-to-go.* Many of my customers tell me that they prepare large amounts of tea at a time and pour it into several water bottles so that they can just reach into the fridge and grab one to go, the same way they would a bottle of water. They carry it around with them all day, sipping steadily. If they're going to be gone for a longer period of time, they take more than one. You can keep the bottle(s) with you all day without being refrigerated; the tea is good to go all day. Most tea is tasty at any temperature, whether it's hot, cold, or room temperature.

* *Be prepared at the office.* Most offices have a coffee station, and many have facilities for heating water and making tea as well. If tea is not supplied, bring your own tea leaves or tea bags, and keep a small pot with a strainer, or just a strainer at your desk. There are many varieties of

strainers available, some that are used for making pots of tea, and some that are good for one cup at a time. If you search online, you're sure to find one that fits your liking. Since you can resteep your leaves several times, you can just keep filling the pot or cup and strainer with hot water and have it available to you all day. If there is a microwave, you can use that as your heat source: heat a cup of water for 30 seconds or the appropriate amount of time according to your microwave, then pour over a strainer of loose tea leaves, or tea bag, into your drinking cup. Save the tea leaves to use again later. Or you can purchase an inexpensive electric immersion heater (a small wand you plug in and place in the cup and it heats the water) so that you can have hot water wherever there is an electrical outlet available.

✸ *Plan when you're out to eat or at a party.* Almost every restaurant in America serves tea today. It may be that they have only one kind of tea to offer—a generic tea bag for all purposes. Or they may have a selection of teas from which to choose. Either way, it's still tea, and you will still get the benefits. And you can always bring your own tea bag and order a cup of hot water. I've done that myself many times. In fact, my advice is to carry tea bags with you wherever you go—in your purse, in your briefcase, in your car. Now, if you are going to a place where there is going to be temptation at every turn make sure you have your trigger or craving tea with you at all times and drink it throughout the event. I have found that instead of feeling I will not fit in because I was not eating all of the fattening foods, everyone was curious as to what I was drinking and why. This has resulted in many an interesting conversation about the tea and its effects. But the key is planning. Bring it and drink it and stay on track.

✸ *Travel with tea.* It's easy to travel with your teas. Pack your favorite teas in any form to have when you arrive along with a small strainer. For the ship, plane, or train, take a few bags or a small amount of loose leaf tea in a plastic bag with a strainer and ask for hot water. Then steep and enjoy your tea throughout your journey. I have made many new friends by sharing my teas with the airline staff and neighbors sitting next to me. It is a great way to break the ice with some interesting people you might otherwise never speak to on your journeys. You can also purchase T-sac Tea Filters (I found them online), which are chlorine- and bleach-free paper bags for use with loose leaf tea, allowing you to make your own tea bags. So you can fill up a few pouches with your favorite flavors of tea and bring them along wherever you go. They come in several different sizes; the larger ones are handy for making pots of hot tea or jugs of iced tea at home or away.

Basically, there is no excuse for you not to have tea with you at all times. Just remember; *"bring it and drink it."* We all know how important it is to keep the body hydrated, especially when you travel—it's an important element of weight loss as well as general health. And as we learned in chapter 4, tea is actually better for you than drinking water.

> *The effect of tea is cooling and as a beverage it is most suitable. It is especially fitting for persons of self-restraint and inner worth.*
>
> LU YU, *The Book of Tea*

TEAmmate Profile

Name: Marsha L.

Age: 48

Total Weight Loss: 11

Total Inches Lost: 7

Favorite Tea: White Peach

I'm a photographer—I work in the film business. That makes it difficult to be on a diet because there's food available all the time. And I had a child a little later in life, at 43. And I put on some weight, and have not been able to successfully remove it. And I'm really active, so I couldn't understand why my weight had plateaued. But then my doctor told me it was hormones and I'm going through menopause. That made me think if I was ever going to lose weight, now would be the time to do it. So I'm fighting hormones, middle age, kids who want to eat junk all the time, film sets that have food everywhere—it's a lot.

The thing that's really changed in my life is the tea. And cooking with tea. Who would have thought that? I mean, I cook with spices all the time, but I didn't think that I'd cook with tea. I use the white tea to cook my vegetables like broccoli and cauliflower. I've used the oolong spice on my chicken and I've used it on my salmon. It was delicious.

I take tea to work with me all the time. I brew the tea, and then I put it into a Camel Pack. It's like a backpack that has a soft water holder in it and you put the tea in it and it stays cold, and you drink it through a straw that's attached. It's really hiking gear, but I use it so I can hold my camera and carry my tea at the same time.

But I like to have it when I come home as well. It's just a nice little ritual, being able to pour it cup by cup. I have beautiful little Japanese teacups that I use, and it's a delicate way to savor the taste of the tea.

And I've started exercising. I live in a canyon, so I'm walking up and down hills.

They call it the "butt burners." My energy has really changed. I think it's because I gave up coffee. And I love the taste of coffee. But now I don't miss it at all. I decided I would give the tea a try, and I love it! I drink decaf tea at night, and it fills me up, so I don't want a snack. You can use the leaves and over and over again, and when I'm done with the tea, I put it in my garden, in my compost. And the garden's doing great!

I do feel it is working for me. I'm losing inches, and I've lost pounds—and it's been very noticeable to my friends. And my husband.

The Ultimate Tea Diet
Meal Plan

In March of 2006, I started going to dr. tea's in Beverly Hills simply because it was a wonderful place to write. I was a serious coffee drinker (four cups or more a day) and hardly ever drank tea. One day, Dr. Tea pointed out that maybe all that coffee wasn't so good for me, and he also mentioned that quitting coffee would actually help me lose some weight. I do exercise, but I'm also a writer, which means I sit at the computer much of the day. I had a good 15 extra pounds on me. My downfall was snacking between meals. Usually something sweet. Dr. Tea suggested I drink some sweet tea instead. Initially, I laughed off his advice, but one day I decided to cut back on my coffee just to see what would happen. I found that I felt much better. Once I quit coffee and started drinking tea all day, I found my snacking went down dramatically. I simply did not want to eat as much.

I've never been really successful going on a diet. However, since Dr. Tea seemed to be right about the snacking, I decided to listen to the rest of his advice about what to eat and how to change my eating habits. In

a little over a month, I lost 12 pounds simply by giving up coffee, fol-
lowing the food plan (although I wasn't perfect by any means) and
drinking Dr. Tea's many varieties of teas and Frosteas (only 20–90
calories) all day long.

JASON N., LOS ANGELES

I know why you bought this book. It's because for years you have been gain-ing weight, losing weight, and gaining it back again. You've tried all the new diets that have come along and probably had success with several of them— while you were "on" the diet. As soon as you went "off" it, you were back to your old habits, and your old weight, once again.

So you picked up this book because you thought that you would give it one more try, and you thought that tea might be the "magic" ingredient you have been looking for all this time.

It is and it isn't.

It is, because of the incredible weight-loss and general health properties it contains. It is the one ingredient that has been missing from all the other di-ets you've tried; yet it is the one ingredient that has been consumed for 4,700 years and has never been a part of any other diet plan. It is the one ingredi-ent you can go right back to when you mess up (and we all mess up). But, as I told you right from the start, tea can't do it all by itself. It's part of a TEAm with a well-balanced diet of proteins, carbs, and healthy fats, along with a moderate amount of exercise. You've read about these components in other diet books, but it's the tea that makes this a winning team.

I, too, am part of a team. I am not a doctor or a nutritionist. I am a pretty good cook, but I'm not a professional chef. So I brought in professionals like nutritionist Christine Bybee and chef Pam Ross to add their extensive knowl-edge and expertise to my knowledge of tea, and together we have developed a program that is easy to follow, well-balanced, and contains recipes infused with tea, delicious enough to please any palate.

So why should I expect you to believe that the Ultimate Tea Diet is differ-ent from any other one you've been on before? I don't. At least not until you give it a try. Not until you start drinking tea and can see for yourself what a difference it makes, just like it did for the TEAmmates you've read about throughout the book (you can read more of their stories in the rest of the book).

Don't make any judgments about this diet until you've been drinking tea for a week or two or three and suddenly realize that you're not as hungry between meals as you used to be, that your cravings for sweets and snacks have almost disappeared because you've found a replacement tea for them, and that you're finding it much easier to control what you put in your mouth.

The science of tea makes it possible—the caffeine/L-theanine/EGCG triad that sends your brain signals to help you feel full. That, in combination with changing your thoughts to change your reality, makes it easy to incorporate the Ultimate Tea Diet as a way of eating and a way of life. It has to be easy, because that's the only way you and I will stick to it!

This is not a new fad diet, one you'll start and then can't stay on. I would never put myself on anything like that, so why would I recommend it to you? I am not going to tell you that you will lose some outlandish number of pounds in four weeks, knowing you will gain them back almost instantly. I am not going to tell you to give up carbs, or to weigh and measure every bite you take. This is a lifestyle change, and it is meant to last your lifetime. I want you to have choices; I want you to enjoy your food and feel satisfied when the meal is over; and above all, I want to bring back the confidence that you lost oh-so-many diets ago.

In order to get there, I do want you to give up some of your old habits, like drinking coffee or diet sodas all day and eating fast food and snacking all night. I'm asking you to practice new healthy habits to put in their place. And I do mean *practice*—repeat these new behaviors over and over until you don't have to think about them anymore. Be mindful of what you are eating. Plan your meals in advance. Drink tea all day.

Experts say that it takes at least twenty-one to twenty-eight repetitions before a behavior becomes a habit. The way you form a habit is to simply do it again and again. In order to form a lifestyle, you have to practice a new lifestyle. Tea, by itself, can begin to change your life. But this is a diet book, not just a "drink tea" book, because I want you to be healthy and feel good about yourself. So I ask you to make a commitment to me, to the Ultimate Tea Diet, and most of all to yourself, that you will see this through. Stick with it for at least four weeks and then see where you are. Take note of how many compliments you get, how many times people say, "You're looking great these days!" Or, "What's different about you?" Be aware of how you feel, and how much more energy you have. Take a good look in the mirror and notice how clear your skin is. Think about how long it's been since you had a craving, how much better you are sleeping at night, and how much more capable you are able of handling the stress in your life. And how many inches you have lost.

Although—and this may sound strange in a diet book—the truth is that I don't care if you're thin. I think you're great the way you are. Your weight goal should not be about the pounds you lose, but about feeling comfortable again in your own skin. And I want you to realize that *it's not all about the scale*. Because it's about the way your clothes fit. It's about the fact that you can walk up a flight of stairs without needing an oxygen tank. It's about the fact that you can run in the yard with your children instead of watching them from a folding chair on the patio. It's about walking into a room and having that bounce in your step that only comes from the confidence within. Think for a moment: When was the last time you felt that way? Yes, the pounds will come off. But I don't want you to be so consumed by a number on a scale that you forget to appreciate the real benefits the Ultimate Tea Diet will bring to your entire life.

However, I do care that you're healthy, and we all know that being overweight presents a plethora of health risks. What I want most of all is for you to feel good and to feel good about yourself. That's why what you'll find here is a commonsense plan to lose weight, get healthy, and begin the process of making changes in your life, one cup of tea at a time.

Guidelines

The meal plan and advice you will find below is based on what has worked for me, and I want to share it with you. These are suggestions for you to follow, not mandates. The meals are healthy and delicious. If you want to eat exactly what you find here, be my guest. If you don't, use these plans as guidelines for serving sizes and calorie counts. Feel free to incorporate any part of it into any other diet plan you may be on. But above all, don't be so concerned with every bite you eat that you forget how to live.

The only two dictums of the Ultimate Tea Diet are: 1) add tea to your day—all day; and 2) say you can lose weight. Sometimes the second part is the more difficult of the two. Remember how powerful your thoughts are. As great as tea is, your thoughts are greater. Your thoughts will move you in the right direction to make the right choices, lose the weight, and keep it off. So go ahead and say it: "I CAN LOSE WEIGHT!" And come back to it for the rest of your life each and every time you have the urge to reach out for your binge or trigger food, or continue eating even if you're exploding. Reach out for your tea instead! The weight will come off. You will feel better about yourself and you will start to take control of your life, just like I did.

The Ultimate Tea Diet Weight-Loss Plan

What We Suggest You Drink:

1. *Drink tea all day every day.* Tea's three ingredients—caffeine, L-theanine, and EGCG—have been proven to decrease your appetite and increase your metabolism to help you lose weight. Have tea in your house, workplace, and car. Carry tea with you at all times. Take brewed tea in your water bottle, or buy ready-made tea drinks (sugar-free). Keep tea bags or a small tin of loose tea and a strainer in your briefcase or purse or in your desk drawer at work. Order tea at breakfast, lunch, or dinner out. Drink tea before, during, and between all meals.

2. *It doesn't matter what kind of tea you drink, as long as it is true tea.* You can drink loose leaf tea or tea brewed from a bag, tea that you've bought from an exclusive tea salon or from your neighborhood grocery store. If you wish to drink a Rooibos or an herbal tea, add a pinch or two of true tea to get the weight-loss and health benefits.

3. *Identify and purchase different teas to replace your snacks, desserts, and binge foods.* Fifteen years ago there weren't anywhere near the choices of teas we have today. I had to make my own craving teas by placing a few chocolate chips and caramel bits in my teapot to replace my candy bar habit. Now, I have provided recipes for different craving teas, like Dr. Tea's Candy Bar, in chapter 11, so you can make them for yourself. I urge you to go to your grocer or tea house and see what teas they have. If they don't carry your favorite dessert or craving tea, ask them to do so. Or go online at www.ultimateteadiet.com or any of the other sites you'll find in Appendix A (page 279) and get the tea you love.

TEASER

Sober Up With Tea

Alcohol yields more calories per gram than carbohydrates. If you choose to have a social drink, have a glass of white wine, which is about 70 calories, as opposed to a margarita, which has about 740 calories! More good news about tea—several studies have shown that while alcohol intoxication produces free radicals that can overwhelm the liver's supply of antioxidants, the EGCG in tea greatly reduces the free radical production and subsequent liver damage.

What We Suggest You Eat

1. *Eat three balanced meals a day, including carbohydrates, protein, and fats.* You can create the illusion of more food by using smaller plates. So for four weeks I want you to put away your oversized dishes and use salad plates and small bowls to eat from. A ¾-cup serving of whole-wheat pasta will look like more than enough on an 8-inch plate, but can appear to be a skimpy serving on a 12-inch plate.

Using an 8-inch salad plate, visualize a balanced meal as follows:

◆ *Half the plate should be covered by good, healthy carbohydrates like fruits, vegetables, and whole grains.* Healthy carbs are those that come from the earth, not from a factory or a processing plant. For example, rice comes from the earth, but when it's processed to remove the hull to make white rice, all the nutrients are removed. That's why brown rice is a better choice. You don't need a carbohydrate counter to keep you from overdoing your carbs—let your taste buds be your guide. If you're having fruit, you can tell that a piece of pineapple is sweeter than a piece of cantaloupe; therefore the pineapple has more carbs. Corn on the cob is sweeter than a radish; therefore the corn has more carbohydrates.

◆ *One quarter of the plate should contain lean protein like poultry, fish, lean beef, egg whites, or tofu.* A serving of protein should be the size of the palm of your hand for women and children, and the size of the palm of your hand up to the first set of knuckles for a man.

◆ *One quarter of the plate should contain green or red vegetables.* See the list of "free" foods below.

◆ *The meal should contain a small amount of a healthy fat,* such as 1 teaspoon of olive oil, 2 tablespoons of light mayonnaise, or 1 tablespoon of low-fat salad dressing (see list below).

2. *If you are going to have a carbohydrate snack, have a protein along with it, and vice versa.* Having a protein? Have a carb alongside. When you combine these two elements, you burn more fat than when you have either one alone. So if you have an apple (carbohydrate) for a snack, have an ounce of low-fat cheese or a tablespoon of peanut butter along with it. If you are going to have a small serving of dessert, have it right after your meal, not hours later. That will prevent your blood sugar from spiking, and stop you from storing the carbs as fat.

3. *If you are at a restaurant, order the leanest meat on the menu, which will most likely be grilled white fish or chicken breast.* Steamed veggies with a small baked potato or a half-cup of steamed brown rice are excellent choices for side dishes for your lean meat. Remember to drink small sips of tea between each bite.

4. *Avoid fast food while on the Ultimate Tea Diet—and most other times as well.* If you must eat while in a rush, we recommend going to a deli or sandwich shop. Order a turkey sandwich on wheat bread without mayonnaise. If you do go to a fast-food restaurant, look for the "healthy menu" and use it.

YOUR LEAN PROTEIN CHOICES INCLUDE:

* Beef, filet mignon
* Cheese, American, fat-free
* Cheese, cottage, low-fat
* Cheese, cottage, fat-free
* Cheese, cream, fat-free
* Cheese, Cheddar, fat-free
* Cheese, mozzarella, fat-free
* Cheese, ricotta, fat-free
* Cheese, soy, Soya Kaas, 98% fat-free
* Cheese, Swiss, fat-free
* Chicken breast, boneless and skinless
* Chicken breast, 98% fat-free deli slices
* Egg Beaters
* Egg whites, All Whites or any brand
* Egg whites, fresh
* Fish, albacore
* Fish, catfish
* Fish, cod
* Fish, flounder
* Fish, haddock

* Fish, halibut
* Fish, herring
* Fish, mahi-mahi
* Fish, monkfish
* Fish, salmon
* Fish, scallops
* Fish, sea bass
* Fish, snapper
* Fish, sole
* Fish, striped bass
* Fish, tuna steak
* Fish, tuna chunk light
* Fish, white fish
* Fish, yellowtail
* Milk, nonfat
* Protein bar, any organic brand, low-fat, moderate carbs
* Protein powder, any type, low-fat, low-carbs
* Shellfish, clams, steamed
* Shellfish, lobster, boiled
* Shellfish mussels, steamed
* Shellfish, oysters
* Shrimp, raw
* Turkey breast, 98% fat-free deli slices
* Turkey ground, 99% fat-free
* Vegetarian, Light Life deli slices
* Vegetarian, Lite Life Smart Dog
* Vegetarian, Boca Burger
* Vegetarian, Harvest Burger
* Vegetarian, low-fat tofu, firm or soft
* Vegetarian, Yves bacon
* Vegetarian, Yves Just Like Ground
* Vegetarian, Yves Pepperoni
* Yogurt, Greek, nonfat

* Yogurt, Greek, low-fat
* Yogurt plain, nonfat
* Yogurt, plain, low-fat

YOUR HEALTHY CARBOHYDRATE CHOICES INCLUDE:

* ½ cup brown rice
* 1 small sweet potato
* ½ cup cooked oatmeal
* ½ cup Cream of Wheat
* ½ cup squash, pumpkin
* Popcorn, Pop Secret 98% fat-free
* 1 small potato

TEASER

Carbs: The Real Story

If you do not eat any carbohydrates at all, as some other diet plans recommend, you may end up burning muscle and not fat. Not good. You may lose weight, but it comes from your muscle (see chapter 9). When you reintroduce carbs into your diet you will gain your weight back, but still have not replaced the muscle. So this time, eat three balanced planned meals a day with *healthy* carbs (not fried foods and potato chips), drink tea all day, and eat a healthy snack if you're hungry.

YOUR HEALTHY FAT CHOICES INCLUDE:

* ¼ small avocado
* 1 teaspoon olive, canola, macadamia nut, sesame, flaxseed oil
* 2 tablespoons ground flaxseed

* ⅛ cup raw nuts (about 11 to 12 nuts)
* 1 tablespoon nut butter (soybean, almond, peanut)
* 1 tablespoon extra virgin olive oil

YOUR "FREE" FOODS INCLUDE:

(The vegetables on the following list contain a negligible amount of carbohydrates per serving of 1 cup raw or ½ cup cooked. For this reason, we encourage you to use as much of these vegetables for a meal or a snack, raw or cooked, without guilt.)

* Alfalfa sprouts
* Arugula
* Asparagus
* Bamboo shoots
* Bean sprouts
* Bok choy
* Broccoli
* Brussel sprouts
* Cabbage
* Cauliflower
* Celery
* Cucumber
* Eggplant
* Endive
* Green beans
* Iceberg, romaine, or any other lettuce
* Kale
* Mushrooms, white
* Mustard greens
* Parsley
* Peppers, green bell
* Peppers, jalapeño
* Peppers, red bell

* Radish
* Sauerkraut
* Spinach
* Tomato
* Turnips
* Watercress
* Zucchini

Here are some additional free items. Where serving sizes are indicated, you may have up to four servings per day:

* Bouillon, broth, consommé, 1 cup
* Catsup, 1 tablespoon
* Club soda/Mineral water/Tonic water
* Dill pickle, 1½ medium
* Flavoring extracts
* Fresh or dried herbs
* Garlic
* Horseradish, 1 tablespoon
* Jam, sugar-free, 1 tablespoon
* Lemon or lime juice
* Mayonnaise, fat-free, 1 tablespoon
* Mustard, 1 tablespoon
* Nondairy creamer, 1 tablespoon
* Nonstick cooking spray
* Pickle relish, 1 tablespoon
* Salad dressing, fat-free or low-fat, 1 tablespoon
* Salsa, ¼ cup
* Sour cream, fat-free; 1 tablespoon
* Soy sauce, low-sodium, 1 tablespoon
* Spices
* Sugar-Free Tea Gum (or any sugar-free gum), 1 piece
* Sugar substitutes (best choices are Splenda and stevia)

✳ Syrup, sugar-free, 1 tablespoon

✳ Taco sauce, 1 tablespoon

✳ Tea

✳ Vinegar (balsamic, rice wine, apple cider, etc.), 1 tablespoon

✳ Water

✳ Worcestershire sauce, 1 tablespoon

Remember, your foods don't all have to be bland to be good for you. Use a tea you love to enhance and even change the flavor of a healthy food, whether it's a carbohydrate like brown rice (substitute brewed tea for the water used to cook the rice) or a protein (season your lean chicken breast with a tea-based rub).

TEASER

Keeping a Food Journal

There is one very valuable tool you can use to help keep you on track, and that is a food journal. It's simply a log of everything you eat during the day. It goes back to the idea of being conscious of what you put in your mouth—if you have to write it down, it somehow keeps you more honest (even if it's only with yourself). Studies have shown that people who keep a detailed eating journal consistently lose 64 percent more weight than those who do not.

The Ultimate Tea Diet 14-Day Eating Plan

The following are suggested menus for the next fourteen days. You will find recipes for most of the dishes in chapter 11. In that chapter, you will also find additional recipes that you may substitute for any of the ones in the meal plan.

All meals are interchangeable. You can eat any meal at any time; for instance, you can eat a breakfast for lunch or a dinner for a midafternoon snack, or have a dessert after lunch. You can also add any of the free foods from the lists on pages 130–32 to any of these meals. All teas, Frosteas and Hot Todteas are interchangeable; if you like the taste of a Frostea and want to serve it hot, it will be delicious either way (and vice versa for Hot Todteas). If you find one in particular you love and want to drink that one all the time, that's fine. If you want to drink a different tea at every meal, that's fine also. It's your choice.

TEASER

Snacking Between Meals

The meal plan has a suggested healthy snack. This does not mean it is mandatory unless your physician or health professional has recommended you eat a healthy snack between meals. If you are hungry between meals, chances are it's because you are in the habit of eating at certain times of the day. Next time you're hungry before meal time, try drinking 8 ounces of tea first. Wait twenty minutes and if you are still hungry, then have one of the healthy snacks with some tea.

DAY 1

Start the day with a cup of tea
Drink as much as you like of the tea(s) you love between meals

Breakfast:

Yogurt Tea Parfait (page 192)
8 to 16 ounces tea

Snack:

Apple Pie Hot Todtea (page 192), served hot or cold, as much as you like, with one tablespoon of fat- and sugar-free whipped topping, or any tea you love

Lunch:

Tea-Grilled (page 193) or Regular Chicken Breast
2 cups your favorite free veggies
½ cup brown rice or Tea Rice (page 193)
2 tablespoons Tea Salad Dressing (page 191)
8 to 16 ounces tea

Snack:

1 cup (8 ounces) edamame (soy beans)
8 to 16 ounces tea

Dinner:

Lettuce-Wrapped Tea Turkey Burger (page 194)
Your choice of free condiments
1 medium corn on the cob
1 slice watermelon
8 to 16 ounces tea

Dessert:

Strawberry Chocolate Mint Tea Frozen Yogurt (page 195) or any tea you love

Drink as much of the tea(s) you love throughout the evening

DAY 2

Start the day with a cup of tea
Drink as much as you like of the tea(s) you love between meals

Breakfast:

Breakfast Tea Burrito (page 195)
Tomato Tea Salsa (page 196)
8 to 16 ounces tea

Snack:

Chocolate Hazelnut Torte Frostea (page 196), as much as you like, with one tablespoon of fat- and sugar-free whipped topping, or any tea you love

Lunch:

Mediterranean Tea Salad (page 197)
1 whole-wheat pita pocket
8 to 16 ounces tea

Snack:

Strawberry yogurt bowl: combine in a bowl one 6-ounce flavored nonfat yogurt,
¼ cup strawberries, and
¼ cup cottage cheese
8 to 16 ounces tea

Dinner:

Lemon Tea Baked Halibut (page 198)
Oven-Roasted Tea Asparagus (page 199)
1 medium baked sweet potato
8 to 16 ounces tea

Dessert:

TEAna Colada Frostea (page 199), served hot or cold, as much as you like, with 1 tablespoon of fat- and sugar-free whipped topping, or any tea you love

Drink as much of the tea(s) you love throughout the evening

DAY 3

Start the day with a cup of tea
Drink as much as you like of the tea(s) you love between meals

Breakfast:

Toasted nutty cinnamon bagel: 1 toasted whole-wheat bagel, spread with
1 tablespoon natural peanut butter and topped with
½ cup low-fat cottage cheese, dusted lightly with cinnamon
8 to 16 ounces tea

Snack:

Blueberry Pie Frostea (page 200), served hot or cold, as much as you like,
or any tea you love

Lunch:

Vegetable Tea Soup (page 201) or any soup
4 ounces cooked skinless chicken breast on the side or added to the
soup
1 whole-wheat pita pocket (4-inch diameter)
8 to 16 ounces tea

Snack:

Hard-boiled eggs and yogurt:
2 hard-boiled eggs
One 6-ounce flavored nonfat yogurt
8 to 16 ounces tea

Dinner:

Turkey Tea Meatloaf (page 202)
¾ cup brown rice or Tea Rice (page 193)
8 to 16 ounces tea

Dessert:

Baked Tea Pears (page 203) with Strawberry-Balsamic Tea Sauce (page
203) with 1 tablespoon of fat- and sugar-free whipped topping, or any
tea you love

Drink as much of the tea(s) you love throughout the evening

DAY 4

Start the day with a cup of tea
Drink as much as you like of the tea(s) you love between meals

Breakfast:

Vegetable Mushroom Tea Frittata (page 204)

2 slices 100% whole-grain toast

2 tablespoons low-sugar fruit jam

8 to 16 ounces tea

Snack:

Ginger Bread Hot Todtea (page 204), served hot or cold, as much as you
like, or any tea you love

Lunch:

Tuna tossed green salad with Tea Salad Dressing:

Mix 2 cups of your favorite free veggies with

2 tablespoons Tea Salad Dressing (page 191) or any low-fat dressing, and

3 ounces tuna fish packed in water or 3 ounces cooked chicken breast

1 whole-wheat pita or 1 slice multigrain bread

8 to 16 ounces tea

Snack:

Mini cottage cheese berry bowl: ½ cup low-fat cottage cheese with

1 cup blueberries or any other berries you love

8 to 16 ounces tea

Dinner:

Tea Chicken Tostadas (page 205)

Tomato Tea Salsa (page 196)

8 to 16 ounces tea

Dessert:

Mint Chocolate Ice Cream Frostea (page 206), served hot or cold, as
much as you like, with 1 tablespoon of fat- and sugar-free whipped
topping, or any tea you love

Drink as much of the tea(s) you love throughout the evening

DAY 5

Start the day with a cup of tea
Drink as much as you like of the tea(s) you love between meals

Breakfast:

Apple-Cinnamon Tea Oatmeal (page 207)
4 scrambled or hard-boiled egg whites
8 to 16 ounces tea

Snack:

Strawberry-Raspberry Pie DaiquirTEA Frostea (page 207), served hot or cold, as much as you like, or any tea you love

Lunch:

Tea Garden Grilled Salmon (page 208)
½ cup brown rice or Tea Rice (page 193)
8 to 16 ounces tea

Snack:

Nutty banana: 1 tablespoon natural almond, peanut, or soybean butter with
1 medium banana
8 to 16 ounces tea

Dinner:

BBQ Tea-Grilled (page 209) or Regular Chicken Breast
1 cup steamed broccoli with fresh lemon juice
1 small baked sweet potato
8 to 16 ounces tea

Dessert:

Tiramisu Rooibos Hot Todtea Tisane (page 209), served hot or cold, as much as you like, with 1 tablespoon of fat- and sugar-free whipped topping, or any tea you love

Drink as much of the tea(s) you love throughout the evening

DAY 6

Start the day with a cup of tea
Drink as much as you like of the tea(s) you love between meals

Breakfast:

1 cup Special K with
½ scoop low-fat, low-carb protein powder
½ cup nonfat milk
¼ cup sliced strawberries
8 to 16 ounces tea

Snack:

1 sugar-free fat-free Popsicle, pudding, or Tea Popsicle (page 210), and
any tea you love

Lunch:

Turkey Sandwich: 2 small slices whole-wheat bread
6 thin slices turkey breast
1 slice fat-free cheese
1 tablespoon light mayo
Any free veggies you desire
1 piece fruit
8 to 16 ounces tea

Snack:

Apple and peanut butter: 1 medium apple with
1 tablespoon natural peanut butter
8 to 16 ounces tea

Dinner:

Tea Chicken Stir-Fry (page 210)
½ cup brown rice or Tea Rice
8 to 16 ounces tea

Dessert:

Orange Sherbet Frostea (page 211), served hot or cold, as much as you
like, or any tea you love

Drink as much of the tea(s) you love throughout the evening

DAY 7

Start the day with a cup of tea
Drink as much as you like of the tea(s) you love between meals

Breakfast:

Fruit Tea Smoothie (page 212)
1 scoop low-fat, low-carb protein powder
8 to 16 ounces tea

Snack:

Caramel-Banana DaiquirTEA/Frostea (page 212), served hot or cold, as
much as you like, or any tea you love

Lunch:

Tea Orange Turkey (page 213) or Tea-Grilled Chicken (page 193)
1 small yam
8 to 16 ounces tea

Snack:

Cheese and crackers: 2 ounces fat-free cheese and
8 fat-free wheat crackers
8 to 16 ounces tea

Dinner:

Tea Chicken Pasta with Sun-Dried Tomatoes and Artichoke (page 213)
8 to 16 ounces tea

Dessert:

Tea-Poached Apricots or Plums (page 214)
Tea Custard Sauce (page 215)
8 to 16 ounces tea

Drink as much of the tea(s) you love throughout the evening

DAY 8

Start the day with a cup of tea

Drink as much as you like of the tea(s) you love between meals

Breakfast:

Egg White Tea Scramble (page 216)

1 slice 100% whole-grain toast spread with

1 tablespoon natural peanut butter

1 tablespoon low-sugar jam

8 to 16 ounces tea

Snack:

Caramel Apple Hot Todtea (page 217), served hot or cold, as much as
you like, or any tea you love

Lunch:

Cold Chicken or Turkey Tea Salad (page 217)

1 slice multigrain bread

1 pear

8 to 16 ounces tea

Snack:

Turkey cheese roll:

1 stick low-fat string cheese rolled up in

1 slice turkey or chicken deli meat

1 pear or apple

8 to 16 ounces tea

Dinner:

Tea Garden Grilled Salmon (page 208)

1 cup Cauliflower Tea Mash (page 218)

1 cup Tea Fruit Salad (page 219)

8 to 16 ounces tea

Dessert:

CappuTEAno Frostea (page 220), served hot or cold, as much as you like, with
1 tablespoon of fat- and sugar-free whipped topping, or any tea you love

Drink as much of the tea(s) you love throughout the evening

DAY 9

Start the day with a cup of tea
Drink as much as you like of the tea(s) you love between meals

Breakfast:

Cheesy toast: 2 ounces fat-free mozzarella over
1 slice whole-wheat toast
One 6-ounce container of nonfat yogurt mixed with
¼ cup fresh strawberries
8 to 16 ounces tea

Snack:

Cinnamon Roast Hot Todtea (page 220), served hot or cold, as much as
you like, or any tea you love

Lunch:

Tea Salad Niçoise (page 221)
1 pear or orange
8 to 16 ounces tea

Snack:

Baked Tea Apple (page 222)
½ cup low-fat cottage cheese or yogurt
8 to 16 ounces tea

Dinner:

Grilled Tea Steak (page 223)
1 cup steamed broccoli
1 small baked potato
8 to 16 ounces tea

Dessert:

Dr. Tea's Candy Bar Black Tea Hot Todtea, served hot or cold, as much as
you like, or any tea you love. (If you're having this tea in the evening
and you don't want the caffeine, don't drink the first steep.)

Drink as much of the tea(s) you love throughout the evening

DAY 10

Start the day with a cup of tea
Drink as much as you like of the tea(s) you love between meals

Breakfast:

Goat (or any low-fat) Cheese Tea Egg Scramble (page 224)
½ grapefruit
8 to 16 ounces tea

Snack:

Chocolate Cream Pie Todtea (page 225), served hot or cold, as much as
    you like, or any tea you love

Lunch:

Tuna stuffed pita: 3.5 ounces water-packed tuna with your favorite free
    veggies
stuffed into a 4-inch whole-wheat pita with
1 tablespoon Tea Salad Dressing (page 191) or any low-fat dressing
8 to 16 ounces tea

Snack:

Fruit and nuts: 12 raw almonds or any raw nuts you love
1 pear or apple
8 to 16 ounces tea

Dinner:

Rosemary Orange Tea Chicken (page 225)
½ cup Tea Rice (page 193)
1 cup cooked spinach
8 to 16 ounces tea

Dessert:

Tea Fruit Salad (page 219) with 1 tablespoon of fat- and sugar-free
    whipped topping, and any tea you love

Drink as much of the tea(s) you love throughout the evening

DAY 11

Start the day with a cup of tea
Drink as much as you like of the tea(s) you love between meals

Breakfast:

Tea-Infused Oatmeal (page 226)
4 scrambled egg whites
8 to 16 ounces tea

Snack:

Vanilla Berry Blast Frostea (page 226), served hot or cold, as much as you
like, or any tea you love

Lunch:

Chef Tea Salad (page 227)
2 tablespoons Tea Salad Dressing (page 191) or any low-fat dressing
1 apple
8 to 16 ounces tea

Snack:

Yam and cottage cheese: 1 small baked yam stuffed with
½ cup low-fat cottage cheese
8 to 16 ounces tea

Dinner:

Tea Chicken Stir-Fry (page 210)
1 cup Tea Rice (page 193)
8 to 16 ounces tea

Dessert:

1 cup sugar-free gelatine or pudding, Tea Popsicle (page 210), or Tea
Fruit Salad (page 219) with 1 tablespoon of fat- and sugar-free whipped
topping, and any tea you love

Drink as much of the tea(s) you love throughout the evening

DAY 12

Start the day with a cup of tea
Drink as much as you like of the tea(s) you love between meals

Breakfast:

Cottage cheese with fruit and nuts: 1 cup of low-fat cottage cheese

1 banana

10 cashews or any raw nuts you love

8 to 16 ounces tea

Snack:

Orange Spice Cake Hot Todtea (page 227), served hot or cold, as much as you like, with one tablespoon of fat- and sugar-free whipped topping, or any tea you love

Lunch:

Chicken or turkey tortilla wrap:

1 whole-wheat tortilla

4 slices deli turkey or chicken

1 slice fat-free cheese, lettuce, tomato, onion or any free veggies, wrapped up tightly

1 apple

8 to 16 ounces tea

Snack:

Protein bar: 1 organic protein bar

8 to 16 ounces tea

Dinner:

Lemon Tea Baked Halibut (page 198)

½ cup Tea Wild Rice (page 229)

1 cup Oven-Roasted Tea Tomatoes (page 228)

8 to 16 ounces tea

Dessert:

Key Lime Pie Frostea (page 229), served hot or cold, as much as you like, or any tea you love

Drink as much of the tea(s) you love throughout the evening

DAY 13

Start the day with a cup of tea
Drink as much as you like of the tea(s) you love between meals

Breakfast:

Breakfast quesadilla:

Two 8-inch whole-wheat tortillas

2 ounces fat-free cheese

2 ounces chicken breast strips and your favorite free veggies, topped with

Tomato Tea Salsa (page 196)

8 to 16 ounces tea

Snack:

Strawberry Pie Green Tea, served hot or cold, as much as you like, with one tablespoon of fat- and sugar-free whipped topping, or any tea you love

Lunch:

Chinese Tea Chicken Salad (page 230)

½ cup steamed brown rice or Tea Rice (page 193)

8 to 16 ounces tea

Snack:

Cheese and popcorn: 1 cup of air-popped low-fat popcorn and

1 stick low-fat string cheese

8 to 16 ounces tea

Dinner:

Tea Turkey Florentine (page 231)

½ cup Tea Rice (page 193)

1 cup green beans

8 to 16 ounces tea

Dessert:

Any fruit you like with Blueberry Tea Sauce (page 231), with 1 tablespoon of fat- and sugar-free whipped topping, and any tea you love

Drink as much of the tea(s) you love throughout the evening

DAY 14

Start the day with a cup of tea
Drink as much as you like of the tea(s) you love between meals

Breakfast:

Waffle with cottage cheese and Tea-Infused Blueberries (page 232)

1 whole-grain frozen waffle topped with

½ cup low-fat cottage cheese

1 cup Tea-Infused Blueberries

8 to 16 ounces tea

Snack:

Pineapple Upside-Down Cake Hot Todtea (page 232), served hot or cold, as much as you like, or any tea you love

Lunch:

Turkey Bacon–Egg Tea Salad Sandwich (page 233)

2 slices 100% whole-grain bread

8 to 16 ounces tea

Snack:

Peanut butter rice cakes: 2 unsalted plain rice cakes spread with

1 tablespoon natural peanut butter

8 to 16 ounces tea

Dinner:

Grilled Tea Marinated Chops (page 234)

1 cup TEABouleh (page 234)

8 to 16 ounces tea

Dessert:

Tea Apple Sauce (page 235), with 1 tablespoon fat- and sugar-free whipped topping and any tea you love

Drink as much of the tea(s) you love throughout the evening

Emergency Snacks to Tide You Over

When you're trying to lose weight, some days will go exactly according to plan. All your meals will be thought out ahead of time and eaten in a timely fashion so that you don't get too hungry in between.

Other days will be more difficult. For whatever reason, you may have to wait long hours between meals. Or you may find yourself stuck in a situation where the only thing you're able to do is grab a quick bite from the deli or grocery store or—oh, no!—a fast-food restaurant. Here are some suggestions:

VEGGIE SNACKS:

* 1 cup cooked fresh asparagus, topped with 1 tablespoon of fresh lemon juice
* 1 cup steamed zucchini squash, topped with ¼ teaspoon of crushed garlic
* 1 cup of skinned and chopped cucumber, topped with 2 tablespoons white rice vinegar
* 1 cup Japanese cucumber, ¼ cup cherry tomatoes, topped with ¼ teaspoon dried oregano and 2 tablespoons rice wine vinegar
* ½ cup chopped red bell pepper and 1 stalk celery
* ½ cup raw cauliflower florets and ½ cup raw broccoli florets, topped with 1 tablespoon fat-free creamy garlic salad dressing

ON-THE-GO GROCERY STORE STOP:

* 4 ounces (½ cup) fat-free cottage cheese, 1 single-serving bag of cheese crackers, such as Pepperidge Farms Goldfish
* 8 pieces tuna sushi
* 1 protein or energy bar—you want the ones with the lowest amount of fat and sugar (10 grams or less), and the highest amount of protein (20 grams or more), 1 small apple
* 1 ounce turkey jerky, 5 dried apricots

FAST FOOD STOPS:

* 6-inch Subway roasted chicken breast sandwich
* 1 soft chicken taco from Taco Bell's "Fresca" menu
* ½ Burger King chicken broiler sandwich without the cheese and mayonnaise

Strategies for Smart Shopping

There are two things you need to start the Ultimate Tea Diet: tea, and a plan. You want to have tea available to you at all times and you want to have a plan (see steps number 2 and 4 from chapter 6) so that every day, you know what you're going to eat and what you need to have at hand in order to fulfill your menu.

That begins, of course, with shopping. A trip to the supermarket can be like a trip to Temptation Island: the aisles are lined with displays designed to lure you in; items you never knew you needed but now you "gotta have" are on sale; check-out areas are lined with candy. If you plan ahead, you can make fewer trips to the market, and fewer trips means less temptation.

Here are some tips for smart shopping:

* Check your refrigerator, freezer, cabinets, and pantry for items you need to stock up on or replenish.

* Plan your meals for the next several days (or for the week) and be sure you have the items you need to make the recipes you have chosen. A 2006 survey showed that by four in the afternoon, almost 80 percent of Americans still don't know what they are having for dinner. If you fall into that group, it usually means fast food, or a quick stop at the grocery when you're tired, hungry, and in a rush to get home—which translates into an impulse buy of something quick and easy and not necessarily nutritious.

* Make a list before you go to the store.

✳ Do not buy your binge or trigger foods; replace them with a similar-tasting tea.

✳ If at all possible, avoid shopping with children or grandchildren. They have mastered the art of persuading you to purchase items that are not on your list, and are usually unhealthy as well (and they really don't need another bag of cookies in the house either). Not only that, you spend 10 to 40 percent more with them along.

✳ Don't shop when you're hungry. You may not make the best judgment on what to get (or how much to get) when your blood sugar is running low.

✳ Stick to the store periphery. Many stores stock their basic staples—fresh fruits and vegetables, breads and other grains, raw meats, seafood, and dairy products—on the periphery of the store. Many premade meals (frozen, canned or dried) tend to be found in the middle aisles. And watch out for the ends of the aisles—that is where the sugar-laden, high-fat snack foods are often found, where they can easily be seen by children.

Read Your Labels

TEASER

If You Can't Read It, Don't Buy It!

Can't understand an ingredient on the label? Don't buy the food. It usually means the addition of chemicals and other items blended from the laboratory that has no place in our diets much less our bodies.

It is amazing how much we buy without knowing exactly what we're getting. That is due, in part, to the fact that it can be difficult to read labels, especially if we don't know just what we're looking for. Remember that ingredients are listed from largest to smallest amounts, and that most nutrition facts are listed *per serving*. That means that a bottled beverage, for instance, may list 40 calories on the label—but that is for one serving, usually 8 ounces, and there can be any number of servings in the bottle, depending on its size.

The Food and Drug Administration has set up guidelines for "nutrient content claims" such as low-fat and low-calorie items. Here are some claims commonly found on food labels and their legal definitions:

✳ Free:

♦ *Calorie-free* means fewer than 5 calories per serving

♦ *Fat-free* (or trans-fat-free) means less than 0.5 grams per serving

♦ *Sugar-free* means no table sugar is in the product. That does not mean it has no calories, and it may still contain natural sugars

✳ Low:

♦ *Low-saturated fat* means 1 gram or less per serving

♦ *Low-fat* means 3 grams or less per serving

♦ *Low-cholesterol* means 20 milligrams or less and 2 grams or less of saturated fat per serving

♦ *Low-sodium* means 140 milligrams or less per serving

♦ *Low-calorie* means 40 calories or less per serving

✳ Lean and Extra Lean:

♦ *Lean* means less than 10 grams of fat and 4.5 grams or less of saturated fat, and less than 95 milligrams of cholesterol per serving

♦ *Extra lean* means less than 5 grams of fat, less than 2 grams of saturated fat, and less than 95 milligrams of cholesterol per serving

TEAhaviors

New behaviors are always difficult at first. It's always easier to start a new habit than to give up an old one. So start by drinking as much tea as you can during the day. Keep tea in your cup, mug, glass, or portable bottle and sip all day; drink with meals; drink in between meals. Make up your own favorite tea drinks to have at any time of day and see how the pounds and inches come off.

You'll then find it much easier to stop eating between meals or late at night. You'll begin to feel better (without experiencing the pains associated with eating less you may have felt on other diets) and want to improve your eating habits to go along with your newfound energy and "alert relaxation" that comes from the tea's L-theanine. Make a commitment to yourself. Plan your meals. Change your reality.

In his book *Mindless Eating: Why We Eat More Than We Think,* author Brian Wansink says that the average person makes well over 200 decisions about food every day. However, about 90 percent of the time we are not even aware of the decisions we make. And much of the time, the reasons we eat more than necessary are due to optical illusions. For instance, Wansink threw a party for some students and served Chex Mix in both gallon bowls and half-gallon bowls. Using scales hidden under a tablecloth, he measured how much each guest took. Students who had served themselves from the gallon bowl took 53 percent more than those who had served themselves from the smaller bowl.

Wansink also recommends dishing out 20 percent less food than you think you want (except for fruits and vegetables—then you should think 20 percent more). Remember, especially in restaurants where you can get oversized servings of food, you don't have to eat everything that's put in front of you. Most people will keep eating until the food on the plate is gone; don't let the empty plate be your signal to stop eating. Let your body tell you when it's full and start to listen. And when you are at home, don't make it easy to overeat. If you're having a snack, for instance, put a serving on a plate, then close the bag or box and put it away at the back of the refrigerator or cabinet. That makes it less convenient to serve yourself a second helping, and you have to make a conscious effort to do so.

I don't expect you to be perfect at every meal. Do the best you can. And go right back to your tea if you do mess up. We have included calorie counts for the recipes in chapter 11, but these are only guidelines. Feel free to try these meals and freely substitute any of them the way you would like them prepared. Nothing will turn you off your good diet intentions faster than eating the same boring meals over and over. Take special notice of the Quick & Easy recipes for those occasions when you are pressed for time but still want something healthy and delicious.

TEASER

Go Organic!

If possible, go organic. Healthy, pure foods taste the best because they offer the best that Mother Nature has provided. Taste buds adjust sweetness levels according to what they are offered regularly. If you provide your body with foods that are not overly processed, your taste buds will learn to appreciate the sweetness of a piece of fruit, for example. It is the processing of food that pulls us farther from true flavor and, simultaneously, pulls us away from the health benefits that food should and can present.

Hippocrates said, "Let food be thy medicine and thy medicine be thy food." Maximize your potential and make every bite count! Eat slowly. Savor each bite. Think about how with each bite, you are improving your health, working toward reaching your goals, and finally caring for yourself.

Tea does our fancy aid,
Repress those vapours which the head invade
And keeps that palace of the soul serene.
EDMUND WALLER, "OF TEA"

TEAmmate Profile

Name: Kate S.
Age: 41
Total Weight Loss: 9
Total Inches Lost: 14
Favorite Tea: Earl Grey

I'm a mother of three. My husband and I own a restaurant, and I was a clothing designer until I had my third child, and then I became a full-time mother. I have always been a pretty active person, and have never been overweight. But since I hit my 40s, I started putting on some weight. So I wanted to lose those 15 pounds I couldn't get rid of.

I was just looking for a diet program, but it became much more of a life change. I went from being a die-hard coffee drinker my whole life to not drinking it at all anymore—with the exception, maybe, of a cappuccino now and again. I just feel like I'm thinking more carefully about what goes into my mind and body. You know, as Dr. Tea says: "If you *say* you can do it, you can do it."

I love drinking the tea. And making the tea—the whole process of brewing it and steeping it—it's like a ritual, almost, in the morning. And it comes out in such a beautiful form when the leaves get wet. I just keep a pot going all day long. It feels very cleansing, and I think my skin's better.

I keep thinking about all the good things those antioxidants are doing for me. Really, it's like a miracle fluid. And for one thing, I sleep better. I was taking a little sleeping pill every night—you know, the over-the-counter kind? I would go to bed with two Motrin and a sleeping pill every night. I stopped that as soon as I started the Ultimate Tea Diet. I haven't had to take any since I started the Diet, and I've been sleeping really well every night.

I work three days at the restaurant, and I drink tea all day. We brew iced tea there, so sometimes I end up drinking that. Otherwise, I have two little pots on the stove. And I will pour a cup, and I just keep refilling it and reusing the same tea leaves all day long. By then all the caffeine is gone, and I can keep drinking it at night.

My children are drinking tea now, too, and they love it. They're 9, 7, and 3. And my husband's been drinking quite a bit, too.

Being in the restaurant business, I love to cook. I have been experimenting with cooking with tea. I've been crushing tea and putting it in everything: cereal, sandwiches, broccoli, pork tenderloin . . . We've used the tea rubs quite a bit, whenever I cook chicken or fish. And I use tea water in rice or to steam vegetables. It's just been a great time to reevaluate what you put in your mouth.

For me, the great thing about this diet is that it's not regimented. It's not saying you have to eat this in the morning, and that for lunch. It gives you basic guidelines for putting meals together. And if you fall off the diet once in a while, you have a cup of tea, and you get going again in the morning.

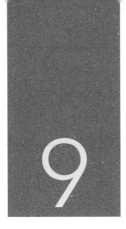

Get Moving:

The Ultimate Tea Diet Exercise Plan

Here's a bold statement: mankind was not built to live in the modern world. We are genetically programmed to be able to move, to hunt for food or to escape from danger. When we shared our habitat with animals in the wild, our physical strength and endurance could mean the difference between life and death.

What we don't realize is that even in the modern world, our physical strength and endurance still mean the difference between life and death. The benefits of exercise, as you'll see in this chapter, can help you live longer, be more productive, and lose weight. However, since we now live in a world of convenience, we have to work a little harder at working harder. It's too easy just to sit on the couch doing nothing, changing the channel, turning on the air conditioning, and lowering the lights by remote control. With trains, planes, and automobiles readily available, we hardly have to walk anywhere anymore. Why, our cars can now even park themselves.

I'm not knocking the modern world. I am a big fan of convenience. However, all of this technological advancement has made us a sedentary society. And it has made more than 60 million of us overweight.

There is no way to get around it—if you want to lose weight, you've got to get moving.

The Benefits of Exercise

Just in case you had any doubts that exercise is good for you, here are some facts that might convince you. Regular physical activity can improve health and reduce the risk of premature death in the following ways:

* *Heart disease and stroke:* Daily physical activity strengthens your heart muscle, lowers your blood pressure, raises your HDL (good) cholesterol levels, lowers your LDL (bad) cholesterol levels, improves blood flow, and reduces the buildup of plaque in arteries.

* *Respiratory health:* Exercise strengthens your lungs as well. Your blood travels through your circulatory system more efficiently, bringing oxygen from your lungs to the rest of your body.

* *Osteoporosis:* Strength training exercises are particularly good to promote bone formation, preserve bone mass, and prevent bone loss. When you strengthen your muscles and bones, you also improve your balance and reduce your risk of falling (extremely important as you get older).

* *Diabetes:* Diabetes is a disease that affects the way your body handles blood sugar. Exercise helps insulin work more efficiently and can help lower blood sugar. According to the Mayo Clinic Web site (www .mayoclinic.com), as your muscles contract during exercise, they use sugar for energy. To meet this energy need, sugar is removed from your blood during and after exercise, which lowers blood sugar levels. Exercise also reduces blood sugar by increasing your sensitivity to insulin, allowing the body to bring more sugar into your cells.

* *Cancer:* Studies have shown that regular exercise helps lower the risk of colon, prostate, uterine, and breast cancers.

* *Sleep:* Moderate exercise at least three hours before bedtime can help you relax and sleep better at night.

* *Stress relief:* Regular exercise activates neurotransmitters including serotonin, norepinephrine, and endorphins—all of which are associated with mood, depression, stress, and anxiety. The levels and balance of these neurotransmitters are important in keeping you on an even keel. If you've had a bad day, there is nothing better to calm you down and lift your mood than to get in a good workout at the gym or to take a brisk walk.

Tea and Exercise

Does any of the information above ring a bell? If you look back at chapters 3 and 4, you will see that tea can also improve health and reduce the risk of premature death from heart disease and stroke, respiratory ailments, osteoporosis, diabetes, cancer, sleep disturbances, and stress and anxiety. That makes tea and exercise quite a powerhouse combination.

In fact, there have been a number of studies that prove that tea actually pumps your exercise benefits up a notch:

* A study published in the *American Journal of Physiology-Regulatory, Integrative and Comparative Physiology* in January 2006 showed that green tea extract increased exercise endurance 24 percent in mice over a ten-week period. Researchers found the tea extracts stimulated the use of fatty acids by muscle, which may help to explain the tea's weight-loss effect. About four cups of tea daily would emulate the effects of the experiment in a human athlete. The effects were not shown after a single use, which led researchers to believe that regular exercise, over an extended period of time combined with tea consumption, enhances the body's ability to "preferentially utilize fats rather than carbohydrates."

✳ A study published in 2005 in *Medicine and Science in Sports and Exercise* set out to explore the effects of dietary supplementation with green tea extract (GTE) and regular exercise on a group of mice that were fed high-fat diets to make them gain weight. The mice were divided into several groups, according to various combinations of GTE and exercise. The results were that after fifteen weeks, GTE alone and regular exercise alone caused a 47 and 24 percent reduction, respectively, in body weight gain induced by the high-fat diet and when combined, resulted in an 89 percent reduction. In the same vein, another study published in the *Journal of Health Science* (2005) aimed to analyze the effects of the combination of regular exercise and tea catechins (antioxidants) intake on energy expenditure. In this study, human beings were the subjects. Divided into two groups, they were given either a beverage containing tea catechins or one without for two months. During this time, they exercised on the treadmill at a set rate for 30 minutes, three times a week. The result? "Fat utilization for energy expenditure under both sedentary and exercising conditions was significantly increased by the combination of regular exercise and tea catechins intake compared to that by exercise alone." That means when the participants were drinking tea and exercising regularly, they were more effectively utilizing fat for energy—even when they were doing nothing at all!

Needless to say, there are many more studies I could cite and many more that are ongoing. The point is that the combination of tea and exercise is proving to be a very effective pairing if you want to make the most of your exercise hours and your weight-loss abilities.

Time to Get Started

Some of you may already be exercising, which is great. And, if you have started drinking tea all day every day, you may already be seeing a difference in your stamina and in your weight loss.

If you are not already exercising, now is the time to get started. The U.S. government Centers for Disease Control (www.cdc.gov) advises that if you are just starting to exercise or if you have been inactive for a while, you should use a sensible approach by starting out slowly. Here are some tips from their Web site:

* Begin by choosing moderate-intensity activities you enjoy the most. By choosing activities you enjoy, you'll be more likely to stick with them.
* Gradually build up the time spent doing the activity by adding a few minutes every few days or so until you can comfortably perform a minimum recommended amount of activity (30 minutes per day).
* As the minimum amount becomes easier, gradually increase either the length of time performing an activity or the intensity of the activity, or both.
* Vary your activities, both for interest and to broaden the range of benefits.
* Explore new physical activities.
* Reward and acknowledge your efforts.

I know what you're saying: "I don't have time to exercise; don't you know how busy I am?" Or: "I'm too old to exercise." Or: "I'm not feeling well today, I'll do it tomorrow." But these are just some of the "I cant's" you've been saying to yourself for a while now. The days pass into weeks, the weeks into months and before long you haven't done anything for years. However, remember my mantra, "If you say you can, you will." If you say you can exercise, you will. Don't give in to the excuses you've always used. Exercise doesn't always have to mean going to the gym or endlessly jogging around the track. You're never too old and you have many opportunities during the course of your everyday life to be more active. For instance:

* Walk to work, school, your place of worship, your nearest store, etc.
* If you drive to your destination, park down the block or at the far end of the parking lot.
* Get off the bus or subway several stops before your destination and walk the rest of the way.
* Take the stairs instead of the elevator or escalator.

* Don't just watch TV—exercise at the same time. Use the treadmill, stationary bike, or stairclimber, or do weight-bearing exercises.
* Join a walking group.
* Take part of your lunchtime and do some walking.
* Play tag with your kids.
* Join a dance class.
* The same way you keep tea with you at all times, keep your walking shoes handy. That way, if you unexpectedly find yourself with free time, you can lace up your sneakers and sneak in a quick walk or run wherever you are.

Essential Fitness: Cardiovascular Exercise

The fat-burning myth that dictates we must be moving fast and furious and end up huffing and puffing in a bucket of sweat in order to lose weight has brought much confusion to exercisers everywhere. Author and philosopher Alfred A. Montapert once said, "Do not confuse motion with progress. A rocking horse keeps moving but does not make any progress." That is the truth when it comes to exercise. Smart exercise is the key to losing weight. Many people think if they are just moving fast, they are making a difference. Unfortunately, exercise must be properly executed or you're just spinning your wheels.

TEASER

A Word of Caution

Before you start any kind of exercise program, you must consult with your physician or health care professional. If you are given the okay, you might want to hire a personal trainer (on your own or at the gym), even if it's for just one or two sessions so that you understand what to do without hurting yourself.

Exercising correctly starts with understanding the two types of exercise: cardiovascular and strength training. Let's talk about cardiovascular exercise first. Cardiovascular (or cardio) exercise works the heart muscle and is the only type of exercise responsible for extreme fat burning.

Here's why: There are two types of muscle fibers in our bodies, slow twitch and fast twitch. Our muscles contain a mixture of both slow and fast fiber types. On average, we have about 50 percent slow and 50 percent fast fibers in most of the muscles used for movement. However, the actual proportion is determined genetically before birth. That's why some people are better at endurance sports, and some are better sprinters.

1. *Slow Twitch (Type 1) the fat burners:* Slow twitch muscle fibers, which appear reddish in color, contract mainly during exercise such as jogging, swimming, bike riding, and brisk walking. The slow twitch fibers are loaded with microscopic cells called mitochondria, within which a cellular metabolic process called the "Krebs Cycle" takes place. The Krebs Cycle is responsible for kick-starting the fat-burning process. Therefore, you will burn mostly fat when using "slow twitch" muscle fibers.

2. *Fast Twitch (Type 2):* Fast twitch fibers are much better at generating short bursts of strength or speed, but fatigue more quickly. Fast twitch muscle fibers contract mainly when intense, fast bursts of energy are needed. For example, when you need to lift a heavy object, punch, kick, sprint, climb up a hill, or do any exercise that requires intense strength, immediately.

Fast twitch muscle fibers are white in color because they do not have as many of those precious little fat-burning mitochondria cells. Glycogen (the form in which foods are stored in the body as energy) within muscle tissue fuels fast twitch muscle fibers. The main source of glycogen is carbohydrates. So if you follow certain fad diets and cut out carbs altogether, your muscles don't get enough glycogen and your body starts to break down muscle tissue which appears as weight loss. This is not the lifetime weight loss we are seeking, because as soon as you reintroduce carbs into your diet, you gain back the weight lost from muscle and the only thing you have accomplished is adding another failed fad diet to your long list of other fad diets that did not work.

Your Target Heart Rate

We now know to burn fat more efficiently during exercise it is important to exercise correctly using your slow twitch muscle fibers. So how do you know which muscle fibers you are using? Many studies have proven that slow twitch muscle fibers contract when you exercise within 65 to 85 percent of your maximum heart rate, or what is called your "target heart rate" zone (THR).

1. The body uses more calories from fat for energy during exercise while in this zone.
2. Exercising in a zone that is too high encourages the muscles to burn more sugar than fat, while reducing energy levels.
3. Exercising in your target heart rate zone is not overly exerting; therefore it allows you to exercise longer than if you were above the high end of your heart rate zone.

In order to calculate your target heart rate (THR), you can use the following formula:

220 – your age = ___ × .65 = ____ the low end of your zone.
220 – your age = ___ × .85 = ____ the high end of your zone.
YOUR TARGET HEART RATE ZONE
_____ (low end) to _____ (high end).

Suppose you are 40 years old. Your formula would look like this:

220 – 40 = 180 × .65 = 117 (the low end of your zone)
220 – 40 = 180 × .85 = 153 (the high end of your zone)

YOUR TARGET HEART RATE ZONE:
117 (low end) to 153 (high end).

The easiest way to keep track of whether you are in your THR zone while exercising is to purchase a heart rate monitor, which you can find at many sporting goods stores or on the Internet. But if you don't want to mess around with any of this just start to do some moving and add to it as it becomes easier.

Exercise Intensity and Duration

If you have been performing cardio on a regular basis, you should continue at that level. If you are just beginning a cardio program, the key is to start slowly and not overdo it. Consult your physician and/or speak to a trainer. The following chart can help you get started (it includes strength training, which you'll learn about next):

DR. TEA'S WORKOUT CHART							
	Day 1	Day 2	Day 3	Day 4	Day 5	Day 6	Day 7
Week	Mon	Tue	Wed	Thurs	Fri	Sat	Sun
1	15 min cardio	Strength 15 min	15 min cardio	off	15 min cardio	Strength 15 min	20 min cardio
2	20 min cardio	Strength 15 min	20 min cardio	off	20 min cardio	Strength 15 min	25 min cardio
3	25 min cardio	Strength 20 min	25 min cardio	off	25 min cardio	Strength 20 min	30 min cardio
4	30 min cardio	Strength 20 min	30 min cardio	off	30 min cardio	Strength 20 min	40 m cardio
5	40 min cardio	Strength 20 min	Continue doing strength and your cardio a minimum of 4 days per week and work up to 60 min per session to maintain your fat loss.				

Your cardiovascular exercise can be performed by using the following: walking on flat land, climbing stairs, treadmill, elliptical trainer, stationary bike, swimming, biking, jogging, or any other form of exercise that involves the large muscles of the hips, thighs, and buttocks.

Exercise Duration and Fuel Burning Ratios

The chart below shows the ratio of fat to sugar burned when you exercise. The longer you exercise within your target heart rate, the more fat you burn (and the more weight and inches you lose).

DURATION	INTENSITY	FAT BURNED	SUGAR BURNED
Rest	None	50%	50%
10 min	THR	40%	60%
20 min	THR	60%	40%
30 min	THR	70%	30%
40 min	THR	75%	25%
50 min	THR	80%	20%
60 min	THR	85%	15%
120 min	THR	99%	1%

Percentage refers to ratio of fat to sugar burned during exercise at target heart rate.

Essential Fitness: Strength Training

The second type of exercise, strength or resistance training—increasing muscle strength by pitting the muscles against a weight or force—is just as important as cardiovascular training, especially as we age and naturally lose muscle mass. Building muscle helps burn more calories. When you burn more calories, fewer calories remain to be stored as body fat. As you lose muscle mass, either from age or lack of use, your capacity to store glucose decreases, your ability to regulate blood sugar levels decreases, and you endlessly wonder to yourself, why am I gaining weight when I'm eating so well? Drinking tea can help ameliorate these processes, but it can't stop them altogether because you're not using as much muscle as you used to do. Resistance training, building and maintaining your muscle mass, is an important key to losing weight, and is particularly important for women because they usually start off with more body fat and less muscle mass than men of the same age and weight.

One very important thing you need to know about exercise: There is no such thing as "spot reduction." Strength training will help you gain strength, not melt fat in one specific area, like your stomach (abs). Cardiovascular exercise is the only form of exercise that melts away fat.

But don't throw the baby out with the bath water. Strength training has a host of benefits and can transform a body when combined with the Ultimate Tea Diet and proper cardiovascular exercise.

First of all, a toned muscular body definitely turns heads. Call me old-fashioned but I still think a person with lean muscles looks much better then a person with a sunken, shriveled body. Second, muscle burns fat all day and night. Your resting metabolic rate (RMR) is the number of calories you will burn in a day at rest. Your RMR increases when your muscle mass increases. What does this mean to you? It means with more muscle you will have a faster metabolism and can burn more fat even while not exercising.

Third, lifting free weights is an energizing and invigorating experience. The strength increase helps make everyday tasks like lifting groceries out of your trunk, carrying your children, or going up a long flight of stairs much easier. Lifting weights has also been known to increase bone mass and density, reducing your risk of osteoporosis. Increased muscle mass can also reduce your risk of injury and speed up recovery if you do get injured.

There are numerous ways to strength train and you should choose what you enjoy most. Pilates, yoga, weight lifting, core training (working the core muscles: abs, buttocks, chest), outdoor exercise courses, body sculpting, and calisthenics are all great ways to train your muscles. Do what you enjoy most and make it a habit two to three times a week. I used to do 15 to 20 minutes of strength training on the off days from my cardio. I had the time, but many of us do not. So you can do some strength training right after your cardio, which is better than doing it before your cardio, because your muscles are already warmed up.

You can never get a cup of tea large enough or a book long enough to suit me.

C. S. LEWIS

TEAmmate Profile

Name: John B.

Age: 34

Total Weight Loss: 19.5

Total Inches Lost: 17

Favorite Tea: Moroccan Mint Green Tea

The biggest change I've noticed is in my energy. Instead of peaks and valleys, I feel like I am more alert and engaged throughout the day. I drink decaf tea at night and it really detoxes me for the following day. I don't feel like I'm in a fog all morning.

I haven't really dieted before. This is my first time. I am thinking about eating differently now. Now it doesn't feel like I am at war with myself wanting to pig out. I make compartmentalized choices for each meal. I am really excited about being a bit more fit. My daughter is walking now and it is nice to be able to chase her around the house and not need to sit down after ten minutes.

I drink tea all the time. Anywhere you go, when you're out and about, you can find tea, hot or cold, fresh or bottled. So I drink it all the time. My wife is very proud of me and my mother-in-law said I looked lighter. My sister did, too. It's nice to hear that stuff, but it's better to feel that way about myself.

What I've learned is that this is a package deal—you have to eat well and you have to exercise as well. It's not just a magic cup of tea and you lose a ton of weight. If you're not doing the work, you're not going to see the results.

But my health is also much improved. I have noticed my asthma is not as prevalent. I'm able to do more cardiovascular exercise now that I'm not carrying as much weight. I had severe intestinal problems last fall because I was drinking coffee. Those symptoms went away when I stopped, but now that I am on tea I feel like my gastrointestinal system is working really well.

When I messed up, I just got back on. I drank more tea. I ate less at the next meal. I worked out harder. I learned to think of it as not messing up as much as tipping the balance one way. When I did that, I had to tip it back the other way.

Put Down That Cup of Coffee:

It's Time to Spill the Beans

Dear Dr. Tea,

My daddy used to say, "Learn from others' strong points to offset one's shortcomings." I now know that daddy's advice was well worth following.

I have been a caffeine addict since my early days growing up in Abilene, Texas when I used to drink a six-pack of Dr Pepper a day. My high school and college years introduced me to the powerful effects coffee can have on the system. Picks you up, keeps you up. Great for those late nights studying or writing that last minute history paper. I never thought about how it had become a necessary part of my life. I never realized that I had, in fact, become a caffeine addict. If I had come to grips with it then, I'm sure I wouldn't have cared or changed anything. I liked the smell. I loved the taste. I lived for the effect it had on me.

As the years progressed, I married, had kids, built my business, all *on the back of my ability to juggle many things due to my endless, bountiful energy. I was wired and I loved it. What I didn't realize was that the caffeine, although it gave me the impetus to do so much, changed who I was. I was too harsh with my wife, I lacked the patience and understanding necessary to be a good father, and my employees hated my brisk manner.*

When my marriage was on the rocks and my kids didn't want much to do with me, I thrust myself into my business. I put in more and more hours, and that eventually cost me my marriage. I hit rock bottom emotionally and decided I needed to seek a different path. I began to read books abut Zen philosophy and Japanese poetry. My outlook on life changed, but obviously something was still missing. I was still addicted to caffeine and no matter how I looked at life philosophically, I was still the same person.

I called upon my ex-wife to help. No one knew me better. I asked her what she thought I needed to help me regain her friendship and reconnect with my kids. Her answer was just four little words: "Get off the coffee!"

Dr. Tea, I must tell you that meeting you has changed my life. I don't know why anyone would pay $300 for fifty minutes with a shrink, when they can spend time with you, talking about life, experiencing the interesting world of teas and herbs, for a whole lot less. My first visit to dr. tea's, if you remember, lasted close to five hours. What I really loved was the education that you provided me. The information regarding the caffeine in coffee versus tea was fascinating. Like how, after the first steep, about 95% of the caffeine is rinsed away, but the bit of information that really knocked me for a loop was about L-theanine, and its ability to inhibit the caffeine stimulation that was destroying my life. That has really had the greatest impact on my life. I feel better and I have found the path that I will stay on for as long as I have a breath left. My tea and me!

I salute you, Dr. Tea. I have thrown my coffee maker away and pass those well-known chain coffee houses by without a thought. You helped me and I will do my part to spread the word. You are at the forefront of the tea revolution and I'm glad I'm on the right side.

Gratefully Yours,
Blake S.

P.S. My ex-wife likes the change. So do my kids. Maybe my story isn't finished. I'll keep you posted.

It wasn't that long ago that cigarette smoking was an accepted everyday practice in our country. When I was growing up, everyone smoked—at home, in restaurants, in movie theaters, on airplanes. Once, as a child, I was hospitalized for asthma, and I can remember my doctor coming into the hospital room smoking a cigarette. Then, all of a sudden, one scientific study after another began to pop up. We began to learn about the harmful effects of cigarette smoke. Eventually, we made significant changes in our attitude about smoking. Warning labels appeared on packages, smoking was banned from airplanes, restaurants, and the workplace, all because we had become educated about the dangers. I believe that caffeine, like cigarettes, will have warning labels one day.

Americans drink over 330 million cups of coffee a day. That means we drink 100,000 cups of coffee every 15 seconds of every day. Just think about that for a moment. That's a lot of caffeine. In fact, many people believe that caffeine is the most widely used legalized drug in the world.

Mother Nature has strategically placed caffeine in the leaves of tea, coffee, and other plants, not to get us up in the morning, but to protect the leaves from insects attempting to feast upon them. The insects will come to the leaf to eat and are repelled by the harsh taste of the caffeine. If they should eat the leaf anyway, their nervous systems go into shock and they fall off the leaf—paralyzed from the caffeine. It's Mother Nature's perfect way of protecting her plants.

What happens when you ingest too much caffeine? Your nervous system, too, goes into a state of shock. You consume your coffee, which is digested in your stomach. The stomach then metabolizes the beverage into the blood system. The blood system with caffeine then races all over your body, eventually gets to the brain, secretes the caffeine into the brain and stimulates the beta brain waves (the ones that put you in the fight-or-flight mode). Your pupils dilate, your heart rate increases, your muscles will tighten, and glucose is released into your blood system in order for you to take care of a perilous situation. You think you are energized. But this is not energy, as Stephen Cherniske, a nutritional biochemist who has more than twenty-five years of academic research and clinical experience in the study of the effects of coffee, and author of *Caffeine Blues: Wake Up to the Hidden Dangers of America's #1 Drug* points out. He says, "While caffeine users may feel more alert, the experience is simply one of increased sensory and motor activity (dilated pupils, increased heart rate, and higher blood pressure)."

Of course, coffee isn't the only beverage that contains caffeine. So do many of the most popular sodas, cocoa, over-the-counter drugs, and the steadily increasing varieties of super-caffeinated energy drinks.

Energy in a Bottle

A report in the April 30, 2007 issue of the *Flint (MI) Journal* titled "Beware of Caffeine in Energy Drinks" warned parents of the danger of the ubiquitous high-caffeine beverages now being marketed heavily to teenagers. According to the article, 31 percent of teens report that they consume energy drinks—and they have more opportunities to do so every year, as more than 500 new energy drinks were launched worldwide in 2006 alone. This is a dangerous trend, as teenagers are more sensitive to the effects of caffeine than adults. They can easily get addicted to the roller-coaster effects of these drinks, and they need to keep drinking them in order to feel normal.

These energy drinks typically contain several times the amount of caffeine found in a can of soda or a cup of coffee. They also contain chemical additives and a lot of sugar, which can exacerbate their addictive qualities. As Dr. Andrew Weil stated in his book *From Chocolate to Morphine: Everything You Need to Know About Mind-Altering Drugs,* "The combination of sugar and caffeine seems to be especially habit forming." And even more alarming, research from the American College of Emergency Physicians found that emergency room visits and poison-center calls are increasing due to caffeine abuse. They tracked calls to the Illinois Poison Center in Chicago for three years and found that more than 250 cases of medical complications arose from caffeine abuse, and that 12 percent of the callers had to be hospitalized. The average age of the callers was 21.

Parents need to help kids avoid the caffeine abuse cycle. Obviously, the earlier they start, the more difficult it will be for them to kick the habit. Let your children know how dangerous these drinks can be when used in excess (as teens are liable to do). Why not introduce them to bottled teas which will give them an energy boost, but will also give them the protection of L-theanine and EGCG? Better yet, why not make their favorite iced tea or Frostea at home and fill a bottle for them to carry during the day?

Caffeine Addiction Is Real

As you all know by now, tea has caffeine in it, too. But as you also know, not only does tea have much less caffeine than coffee, but L-theanine counters the effect of the caffeine that it does contain. Coffee, sodas, cocoa and energy drinks do not have any L-theanine. You can see in the chart below how much caffeine tea has in the first steep compared to a regular cup of coffee:

Black Tea	*50 percent less caffeine*
Oolong Tea	*70 percent less caffeine*
Green Tea	*80 percent less caffeine*
White Tea	*90 percent less caffeine*
Rooibos Tisane	*no caffeine (naturally decaffeinated)*

Caffeine is very soluble and is secreted from coffee, tea, and cocoa in the first steep or brew by the addition of the hot water. Tea is the only one of these beverages that you can resteep or brew over and over again; in fact, the second and third steeps are considered to be the best by tea experts. The second steep is 94 to 98 percent caffeine free and any additional steeps are totally caffeine free. You would never resteep your coffee grounds or cocoa drinks because there is no flavor left after the first steep.

Small amounts of caffeine every day won't cause you great harm. I'm not saying that you must cut out every bit of caffeine from your diet, or that you can never have a cup of coffee or can of cola again. I live in the real world, and so do you, so if you enjoy an occasional cup of coffee or can of soda like I do, then go for it—as long as you're drinking it because you *want* it, not because you need it to feed your addiction.

And caffeine is addictive. One of the hallmarks of addiction is that you initially feel "high" from the addictive substance (whether it is a drug like heroin or cocaine, or an activity like gambling or shopping), and then "come down" when that high wears off.

TEASER

I Need My Morning Coffee

That first cup of coffee in the morning seems to be the one people have the most difficulty giving up. So here's my advice: As soon as possible after you have your coffee, drink a cup of tea. That way, you're introducing L-theanine into your system, which will counter the harmful effects of the caffeine. After I appeared on a radio program with Dr. Michael Roizen, author of *You: The Owner's Manual* and *You: On a Diet*, he not only agreed with this philosophy, he said that he would immediately begin incorporating this regime into his daily life.

The Coffee Controversy

There is an ongoing debate in the scientific community about coffee and whether or not it is harmful to your health. As of today, there have been more than 20,000 studies done—and no consensus reached. Several studies have shown that drinking a few cups of coffee a day is actually good for you. Some benefits researchers have found include:

* A lower risk of type 2 diabetes
* A reduced risk of Parkinson's disease
* A reduced risk of liver damage in people at high risk of liver disease
* A 50 percent lower risk of developing gallstones

However, other studies have uncovered associated health risks. Coffee:

* Traps body fat.
* Increases stress.
* Causes insomnia, anxiety, and irritability.
* Causes heartburn and indigestion.
* Increases cholesterol levels in people who drink unfiltered coffee (which includes espresso and espresso drinks).
* Contributes to an increased risk of osteoporosis in postmenopausal women.
* Contributes to a worsening of PMS symptoms in some women.
* Reduces fertility in women trying to conceive.
* Increases blood pressure.
* Raises blood sugars.
* Slows down metabolism.
* Negatively affects sleep, which can increase your appetite.
* Leads to higher levels of inflammatory substances that have been linked to heart attacks and stroke.

In 2002, Dr. James D. Lane, a researcher at Duke University Medical School, told CBS News that he believes the consumption of caffeine probably creates a public health risk because after fifteen years of study, his research showed that "caffeine always raises blood pressure." He also believes that many Americans drink enough coffee each day to raise their risk of heart attack or stroke by 20 to 30 percent. "Half of the adult population of the United States are regular coffee drinkers . . . drinking an average of three to four cups of coffee a day," he said. "That might be 100 million people who are putting themselves at great risk of a heart attack, a stroke, or early death as a result of the coffee drinking they do."

And when it comes to losing weight, coffee comes up short again. There have been a number of studies that prove that coffee has organic acids that raise your blood sugar and insulin. According to the Canadian Diabetes Association, "drinking caffeine in large amounts as coffee over a short period of time has been shown to raise blood sugar. Caffeine does this by enhancing the effect of two hormones (adrenaline and glucagon). These two hormones release stored sugar from the liver resulting in high blood sugar." In response, large amounts of insulin are released into the bloodstream. And, as we learned in chapter 3, when there's high blood sugar, insulin begins to do its job, which is to escort glucose into the liver and muscles where it's turned into glycogen and waits to be burned as energy. If there's more glucose (blood sugar) than there is cell storage space, the excess is converted into fat.

In his book *The Perricone Prescription,* Dr. Nicholas Perricone states that "coffee raises the levels of cortisol and insulin, hormones that accelerate aging and store body fat. Substitute green tea instead, which . . . can also block the absorption of bad fats by 30 percent." He clarified this even further on a November 10, 2004 *Oprah Winfrey Show* appearance, saying that "insulin puts a lock on body fat. When you switch over to green tea, you will drop your insulin levels, and body fat will fall very rapidly."

Canadian researchers have also found that coffee may actually slow down metabolism. Professors Terry Graham and Lindsay Robinson, of the Department of Human Biology and Nutritional Sciences at the University of Guelph, studied the effects of caffeine following a typical breakfast of milk and cereal. For the study, ten healthy male participants aged 20 to 27 were given either caffeinated coffee, decaffeinated coffee, or water, along with a serving of cereal and milk. Following breakfast, all of the participants' blood glucose (sugar) levels rose as they digested the meal. But the caffeinated coffee drinkers released much more insulin than other participants. In theory, the large amount of insulin released in the body should have caused the glucose levels to drop quickly. But three hours later, the glucose levels of the coffee drinkers had still not returned to normal. This suggests that caffeine reduces insulin's effectiveness, and we already know this increases the chances of storing more fat in your cells (and as we know from chapter 3, tea increases your insulin effectiveness).

TEASER

If You Want to Lose Weight, Don't Let Caffeine Keep You Awake!

When your caffeine intake interferes with your sleep patterns, you could be in deep trouble. Sleep deprivation is epidemic in our society. Animal studies have shown that this can be fatal, and it's no different for human beings. And there's now evidence that how much sleep you get could be one of the most important factors influencing weight loss.

Research has recently shown that sleep has an important effect on two hormones that impact our weight: leptin and gherlin. Leptin affects your level of satisfaction after eating a meal. When you don't get enough sleep, leptin levels go down, and when you wake up, you don't feel satisfied after you eat, and we all know what that means— we eat more. At the same time, lack of sleep causes levels of gherlin to rise, which stimulates your appetite. So when you're not sleeping well, you end up eating more food and finding it less satisfying.

The Myth of Decaffeination

Despite what most marketers would like you to think, there really is no such thing as a decaffeinated drink. Even decaffeinated tea contains small amounts of caffeine (tempered, of course, by the L-theanine). However, the amounts of caffeine in "decaf" coffee can vary widely and add up quickly. An October 2006 study published in the *Journal of Analytical Toxicology* stated that "Patients vulnerable to caffeine effects should be advised that caffeine may be present in coffees purported to be decaffeinated." The study's authors found that decaffeinated beverages "are known to contain caffeine in varying amounts." The first phase of the study looked at ten decaffeinated samples from various coffee shops: findings there showed caffeine in the range from zero to 13.9 milligrams per 16-ounce serving. In phase two of the study, "Starbucks espresso decaffeinated . . . and Starbucks brewed decaffeinated coffee . . . samples were collected from the same outlet to evaluate variability of caffeine content of the same drink . . . The caffeine content for the Starbucks decaffeinated espresso and brewed samples collected from the same outlet were 3.0 to 15.8 mg per shot of decaf espresso and 12.0 to 13.4 mg per 16-ounce serving of the decaf brewed, respectively." A 16-ounce cup of regular Starbucks coffee contains about 372 mg of caffeine, and a shot (about 2 ounces) of espresso about 100.

The conclusion? The authors felt that "further exploration is merited for the possible physical dependence potential of low doses of caffeine such as those concentrations found in decaffeinated coffee."

Are You Addicted?

Now that you know what coffee and caffeine consumption does to your body's systems, it might be useful to know just how much caffeine you are consuming on a daily basis. It is sometimes difficult to calculate, because although caffeine added to food and beverages in the United States must be listed as an ingredient, manufacturers are not required to list amounts (although that may be changing in the near future).

The chart below gives you an approximate idea of the caffeine content of some common beverages (these numbers are estimates—no two sources quote exactly the same numbers):

Beverage	Ounces per Serving	Milligrams of Caffeine
7-UP	12	0
A&W Cream Soda	12	29
Amp	8.4	80
Arizona Green Tea Energy	16	100
Barq's Root Bear	12	23
Black tea	8	40–50
Black tea, decaffeinated	8	4
Chocolate milk	8	5
Coca-Cola Classic	12	34
Coca-Cola Zero	12	35
Coffee, brewed	8	80–135
Coffee, decaffeinated brewed	8	5–15
Coffee, drip	8	115–175
Coffee, espresso	2	100
Coffee, instant	8	65–100
Diet A&W Cream Soda	12	22
Diet Barq's Root Beer	12	0
Diet Coke	12	45
Diet Dr Pepper	12	41
Diet Mountain Dew	12	55
Diet Pepsi-Cola	12	37
Diet RC Cola	12	43
Diet Sunkist Orange	12	42
Dr Pepper	12	41
Enviga	12	100
Fresca	12	0
Green tea	8	20–30
Green tea, decaffeinated	8	4
Jolt	12	71
Lipton Iced Teas	20	50
McDonald's large coffee	16	145
McDonald's small coffee	12	109
Minute Maid Orange Soda	12	0
Mountain Dew	12	55
Nestea Iced Tea	16	34
Oolong tea	8	25–30
Pepsi One	12	100

Beverage	Ounces per Serving	Milligrams of Caffeine
Pepsi-Cola	12	38
Red Bull	8.5	80
Rockstar	16	150
Royal Crown Cola	12	43
Sierra Mist	12	0
Snapple Tea	12	32
Sprite	12	0
Starbucks Grande caffe latte	16	116
Starbucks Grande cappuccino	16	116
Starbucks Grande coffee	16	372
Sunkist Orange Soda	12	41
Tab	12	46
White tea	8	10–20

Here are some caffeine amounts you may not think about—many medications contain caffeine. If you're counting daily totals, you should take these into consideration as well:

Product	Tablet	Milligrams of Caffeine
Anacin	1	32
Dristan	1	16
Dexatrim	1	200
Excedrin	1	65
Midol	1	32
No-Doz	1	100
Vivarin	1	200
Vanquish	1	33

Sources: American Beverage Association; US Food and Drug Association; www.mayoclinic.com; www.energyfiend.com

Take the Caffeine Quiz

Using the chart below, fill in the amount of caffeine you consume in a day. Be sure to consider how many servings of each substance you consume. While a cup of coffee or tea is about eight ounces, for instance, a mug may hold 12 or 14 ounces. And we all know that what they call a "small" soda at the movie theater is a true misnomer. Also, remember that if you resteep your tea leaves, each new cup has virtually no caffeine and should be calculated as zero.

When you have filled in the blanks, add up your caffeine consumption score for the day.

Here's a sample chart of the amount of caffeine I was consuming fifteen years ago:

Caffeinated Beverage, Food, or Drug	Number of Servings	Serving Size	Total Milligrams of Caffeine
Black tea	0	8oz	0
Coffee, brewed	15	8oz	1500
Starbucks Grande coffee	1	16oz	372
Diet Coke	1	12oz	45
Excedrin	2	2 tablets	260
Total for the Day:			2,177 WOW!

NOW FILL IN YOUR OWN CHART:

Caffeinated Beverage, Food, or Drug	Number of Servings	Serving Size	Total Milligrams of Caffeine
Total for the Day:			

While no one knows exactly how much caffeine is too much, most experts agree that more than 300 milligrams a day (which is about the equivalent of three cups of coffee) can start to cause you physical problems, including sleeplessness, headaches, muscle tremors, digestive problems, heart palpitation, irritability, and anxiety. Once you get up to the 500 to 600 milligrams per day range, you're most likely addicted (and it's easy enough to do, as you can see from the sample chart). Be aware that different people react differently. Some people are particularly sensitive to caffeine and will start to feel its effects with as little as 100 milligrams a day. When you get above 600 milligrams per day, you may be in trouble. Your risk of heart attack may be more than double that of someone who does not use caffeine, and you're also at risk for a stroke. It's definitely time to cut back, and start your journey towards good health one cup of tea at a time!

We had a kettle; we let it leak:
Our not repairing made it worse.
We haven't had any tea for a week . . .
The bottom is out of the Universe.
RUDYARD KIPLING

TEAmmate Profile

Name: Debbie D.
Age: 40
Total Weight Loss: 10
Total Inches Lost: 16.25
Favorite Tea: Green Tea

I decided to do this program because I've been having a difficult time lately and I needed to do something for myself. Back in November I had a bad fall and broke five bones in my foot. I had to have surgery to have pins put in my foot. So I was on crutches for two and a half months. I just got the pins out in January and started walking again without crutches, with just a boot. As I started doing the physical therapy on my foot, I realized I'd gotten really out of shape and gained all this weight because I hadn't been able to exercise. And so I had started exercising, and then I heard about the tea diet. And then I lost my grandfather recently, and it was a really stressful three weeks of him being ill and us not knowing what was going on. And then my kids had spring break, and we went on a planned trip to Disneyland.

And the one consistent thing that I really stuck to was making my tea.

I took my tea with me. I bought this portable electric water heater, and I made my tea in our hotel room at Disneyland. Through everything, I had my tea with me. And I think it's kept me in a balanced state through all the stress I've been through. And even though there were a couple weeks where my weight fluctuated, I've definitely lost pounds and inches.

I've really been eating a lot better and I've really been making a conscious effort to be aware of what I'm eating when I'm emotionally upset. And I now cook a lot with tea. I add green tea to my vegetables and whatever I'm cooking. We had halibut and shrimp for Mother's Day, and I put green tea in that. And I use oolong tea in my salad dressing.

My kids love the tea. I've bought them some blueberry white tea and peach white tea, and they adore it. I just pour off the first pot so there's no caffeine. I've now stocked my office with a teapot, strainer, and tea, and a lot of my colleagues are starting to drink it.

And now that my foot is better, I've started doing the treadmill five days a week. Even if I can only get on fifteen minutes here or thirty minutes there, I think that's made a huge difference. And it's kept my stress level and anxiety down, as well. Even with all the setbacks I've had, I still continue to lose. And it's not like I spiraled downward and gained weight, which has always happened before when I was on a diet. It seems that I've found better ways to deal with the stress. And I won't say I've eaten perfectly—I've had a bad day here or there. But I've kind of been able to reflect on it and go: "You know, that just didn't work for me." But Dr. Tea always tells us it doesn't matter if you're not perfect. You're already a success. It's not like other diets I've been on that are so strict, where you have to follow the plan exactly or you feel like you're a failure. With the Ultimate Tea Diet, I feel there's a lot of freedom. And I think that's what's worked for me. I think it's really important that even though I may have slid a little bit here and there, just drinking the tea really kept me on track. Instead of making excuses because this or that happened in my life, I've been able to say, okay, this did happen, and I slipped a little bit, but all I need to do to start again is have another cup of tea.

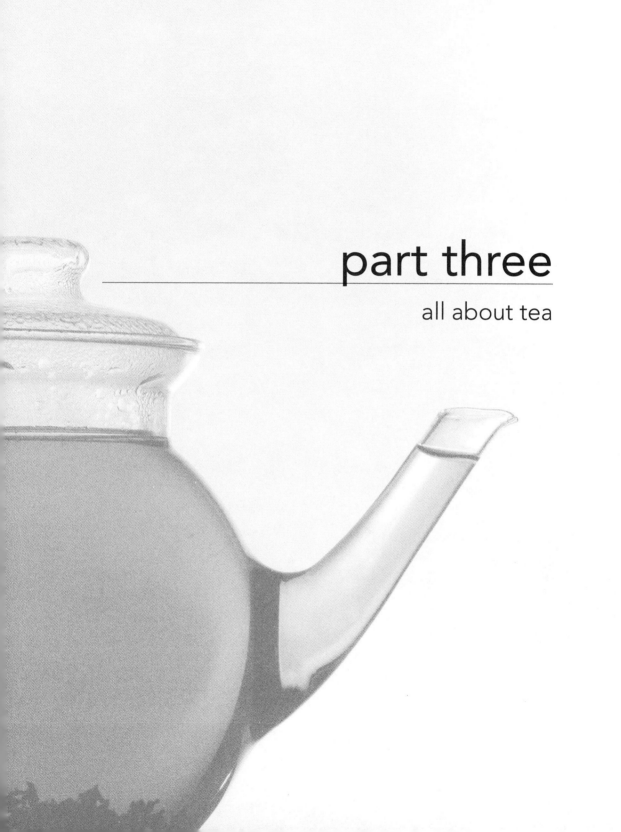

part three

all about tea

11

Dr. Tea's Kitchen:

Tips, Techniques, and Recipes
for Cooking with Tea

The one ingredient you will find in these recipes that you will not find in any other diet is *tea*. All the recipes in this chapter are made with tea. The chapter is divided into five parts:

✳ *Part 1: Rubs and Dressings.* These can be used as seasonings and dressings on any recipes you choose.

✳ *Part 2: Meal Plan Recipes.* These are the recipes for the meals in the 14-day meal plan found in chapter 8.

✳ *Part 3: Quick & Easy Recipes.* We know that you are sometimes limited in the amount of time you have to prepare meals for yourself and your family. That's why we've included recipes that have familiar ingredients and take only a short time to put together. But don't worry, they're still healthy and delicious.

* *Part 4: Additional Recipes.* The dishes here can be substituted for any of the dishes in the 14-day meal plan. We included these recipes so that you won't get bored having the same meals over and over again.

* *Part 5: A Dinner Party for Four with Tea Pairings.* If you're planning a party or special occasion, you can use this menu verbatim or as a guide to a fantastic feast for you and your guests.

When I first started telling my dr. tea's customers about cooking with tea, they looked at me as if I were a mad scientist. What do you mean, cooking with tea? They were a bit less skeptical when I told that them that tea will tenderize your meat, add more flavor to your sauces, and spice up any dish you can imagine. It is, more than anything, a flavor enhancer—it brings out the best from the proteins, carbs, and fats you are already using to lose weight, and adds the Tea3 properties that will aid the process even more.

I promise, there is nothing to be afraid of. I know that some of you are having a hard time with the concept of "eating" tea. But it is perfectly edible. If you really wanted to, you could take loose leaf tea right out of the tin or the bag and eat it. It would do you no harm. But if a recipe calls for "1 teaspoon dry oolong tea," you can use it as is, grind it up into smaller pieces, or just crush between your fingers. If you choose to grind the tea, then it would reduce to ¼ to ½ teaspoon of tea.

Don't be afraid to experiment with your own recipes as well. Just remember that tea brings out the saltiness in food, so most recipes that include tea do not need additional salt.

When you read the recipes, you will see that we have made suggestions for the type of tea to use. (It does not matter which brand you use or if it comes from a tea bag or is loose.) However, feel free to experiment. The tea flavor does not overwhelm any of the dishes, but if you prefer a slightly different taste, use the tea you like best.

Tea seems to bring out the best in everyone and everything! The tea does more than add flavor, however. When you cook the Ultimate Tea Diet way, all the health benefits that come in a cup of tea are now being cooked into your food as well.

PART 1 ✳ RUBS AND DRESSINGS

You may use loose leaf tea or remove the tea from your tea bags. Do not worry about being precise as to the measure of tea, as a little more will only serve to add more health to your dish.

A rub is just what it sounds like: a combination of dry seasonings that you rub into beef, pork, chicken, or fish to bring out the true flavor of the dish. To use a rub, you first spread a very small amount of olive oil onto your meat, rub it in, and then "rub the rub" onto the meat as well. You can do this immediately prior to cooking, but if you want the flavor to permeate and tenderize the meat, you can let it stand for at least 30 minutes (refrigerated overnight is fine, too). Store any leftover rub or dressing in a tightly closed jar.

You can also use these rubs as seasonings for vegetables, salads, and omelets—just sprinkle them on as you would salt and pepper. And don't be afraid to mix and match. If you like to use the chicken rub on steak or fish, go right ahead. They're all tea-riffic!

Chicken Tea Rub

> 2 teaspoons ground black pepper
>
> 1 teaspoon dried thyme
>
> 1 teaspoon kosher salt
>
> 1 teaspoon finely ground dry Plum Oolong Tea, or any oolong tea you love

Mix all ingredients together. Sprinkle lightly on skinless, boneless chicken breasts. May be used more liberally on whole chickens.

Makes 5 teaspoons

NUTRITION PER ROUNDED 1-TEASPOON SERVING: *calories 5, fat 0g, protein 0g, carb 1g*

All-Purpose Fish/Vegetable Tea Rub

4 teaspoons ground white pepper

2 teaspoons kosher salt

2 teaspoons finely ground dry oolong tea

Mix all ingredients together. Use generously.

Makes 8 teaspoons

NUTRITION PER ¾-TEASPOON SERVING: *calories 10, fat 0 g, protein 1 g, carb 2 g*

Steak Tea Rub

4 teaspoons ground black pepper

4 teaspoons chili powder

4 teaspoons packed light or dark brown sugar

2 teaspoons finely ground dry oolong tea

2 teaspoons kosher salt

1 teaspoon paprika

Mix all ingredients together. Use generously.

Makes about 6 tablespoons

NUTRITION PER 1¼-TEASPOON SERVING: *calories 20, fat 0 g, protein 1 g, carb 4 g*

BBQ Tea Rub

4 teaspoons ground black pepper

4 teaspoons chili powder

4 teaspoons packed light or dark brown sugar

2 teaspoons finely ground dry Lapsong Souchong Black Tea

2 teaspoons kosher salt

1 teaspoon paprika

Mix all ingredients together. Use generously.

Makes about 6 tablespoons

NUTRITION PER 1¼-TEASPOON SERVING: *calories 25, fat 0 g, protein 1 g, carb 5 g*

Tea Salad Dressing

> 1 tablespoon olive oil
>
> 2 tablespoons balsamic vinegar
>
> ¼ teaspoon ground black pepper
>
> Pinch of finely ground dry Green Tea
>
> ½ teaspoon Dijon mustard

Mix in a small bowl and drizzle over salad.

Serves 2

NUTRITION PER SERVING: *calories 70, fat 7 g, protein 0 g, carb 2 g*

Tea Tomato-Seed Salad Dressing

> 2 large tomatoes (try to use organic if possible)
>
> 2 tablespoons red wine vinegar
>
> ½ teaspoon dry green tea
>
> ¼ teaspoon salt
>
> ¼ teaspoon ground pepper

Clean and dry the tomatoes. Quarter the tomatoes and remove the seeds with a spoon, placing the seeds into a small bowl. Use the quartered tomatoes for your salad or as a side dish to your breakfast, lunch or dinner.

Combine the tomato seeds, vinegar, dry tea, salt, and pepper and mix. Spoon onto salad or over tomatoes.

Serves 2

NUTRITION PER SERVING: *calories 35, fat 0 g, protein 2 g, carb 7 g*

PART 2 ✳ MEAL PLAN RECIPES

DAY 1

Yogurt Tea Parfait

¼ cup low-fat granola

¼ teaspoon finely ground dry fruit tea or tisane (your favorite)

One 7-ounce container low-fat Greek yogurt

1 tablespoon honey or agave nectar

¼ cup fresh raspberries

2 walnuts, crushed

Combine all the ingredients in bowl, or layer for a parfait effect: pour the granola into a bowl or parfait glass, add the tea, and mix. Combine the yogurt with the honey and spoon half over the granola/tea mixture. Spread the raspberries as the next layer. Add the rest of the yogurt, and sprinkle the crushed walnuts on top.

Serves 1

NUTRITION PER SERVING: *calories 320, fat 4.5 g, protein 21 g, carb 52 g*

Apple Pie Hot Todtea

Apple Pie Black Tea or Rooibos tisane* to cover the bottom of a teapot, or one bag apple-flavored tea

1 teaspoon agave nectar or any honey, mixed with 1 tablespoon hot water

1 cup filtered water

1 tablespoon fat- and sugar-free whipped topping (optional)

Combine the tea and agave nectar in a teapot or cup. Add the water and steep for 3 to 4 minutes, strain, and serve hot with whipped topping, if desired.

*If you do not have the Apple Pie Black Tea or Rooibos tisane, use any plain Black Tea or Rooibos tisane and add 1 teaspoon cubed, peeled dried or fresh apples, a dash of ground cinnamon, and ¼ teaspoon vanilla extract (optional) to the steeping.

If you desire a Frostea, strain the brewed tea over ice in a blender and blend to your desired thickness. Serve with whipped topping, if desired. Resteep the loose or bagged tea.

Serves 1
NUTRITION PER SERVING: *calories 40, fat 0 g, protein 1 g, carb 8 g*
WITH 1 TABLESPOON SUGAR-FREE WHIPPED TOPPING: *calories 45, fat 0 g, protein 1 g, carb 10 g*

Tea-Grilled Chicken

> *Four 4-ounce skinless, boneless chicken breast halves*
> *1 tablespoon olive oil*
> *1 tablespoon balsamic vinegar*
> *2 teaspoons Chicken Tea Rub (page 189), or add ¼ teaspoon finely ground dry tea to your best chicken seasoning*

Wash and pat dry the chicken breasts. Mix the oil and vinegar and rub into the chicken. Sprinkle lightly with chicken seasoning. Allow to sit for 10 minutes.

Heat a grill pan to high. Grill the chicken breasts until well browned.

Serves 4
NUTRITION PER SERVING: *calories 160, fat 5 g, protein 27 g, carb 1 g*

Tea Rice

> *2 teaspoons dry Plum Oolong Tea or other dry oolong tea you love*
> *2 cups boiling water*
> *½ teaspoon kosher salt*
> *½ teaspoon ground black pepper*
> *1 cup brown rice*

Brew the dry tea in the boiling water for 10 minutes (you can still resteep these leaves and use again). Strain the tea into a saucepan. Bring the tea to a boil. Add the salt and pepper. Rinse the rice well. Add the rice to the boiling tea. Lower the heat until tea is at a simmer. Cover the saucepan with a tight-fitting lid and simmer for approximately 40 minutes, or until tea has been absorbed. Fluff with a fork.

Serves 6

NUTRITION PER ½-CUP SERVING: *calories 180, fat 1.5 g, protein 4 g, carb 38 g*

Lettuce-Wrapped Tea Turkey Burgers

1 pound ground white meat turkey

2 eggs

2 tablespoons chopped celery

2 tablespoons finely chopped sun-dried tomatoes

2 tablespoons grated fat-free Parmesan cheese

1 tablespoon chopped fresh flat-leaf parsley or 1 teaspoon dried

2 tablespoons Worcestershire sauce

1 teaspoon finely ground dry green tea

1 teaspoon ground black pepper

½ teaspoon hot sauce

¼ cup panko (Japanese bread crumbs)

Olive oil cooking spray

1 head butter lettuce, leaves separated, rinsed, and dried

Combine the turkey, eggs, celery, tomatoes, cheese, parsley, Worcestershire, dry tea, hot sauce, and panko in a medium bowl, mixing lightly until all ingredients are incorporated. Divide into four portions and form into patties. Heat a grill pan or barbeque to medium. Spray the pan or grate with a little olive oil cooking spray. Cook for about 8 minutes each side.

Serve in the lettuce leaves.

Serves 4

NUTRITION PER SERVING: *calories 210, fat 2.5 g, protein 35 g, carb 13 g*

Strawberry Chocolate Mint Tea Frozen Yogurt

½ cup filtered water

3 tablespoons dry Mint Chocolate Chip Ice Cream Rooibos, or any dry
chocolate tea

1 quart plain nonfat yogurt

1 cup sugar-free frozen strawberries

Bring the filtered water to a boil and remove from the heat. Add the dry tea and steep for 5 to 7 minutes. Strain the tea into a blender or food processor. Add yogurt and strawberries to the tea mixture, and blend until smooth. Place into a freezer-safe container and freeze for 2 hours, or until you are ready to serve.

Makes about 1 quart; serves 4

NUTRITION PER 1¼-CUP SERVING: *calories 120, fat 0 g, protein 13 g, carb 22 g*

DAY 2

Breakfast Tea Burrito

Olive oil cooking spray

½ red bell pepper, chopped

½ yellow bell pepper, chopped

12 egg whites

1 tablespoon chopped cilantro

¼ teaspoon black pepper

⅛ teaspoon finely ground dry oolong tea

Two 8-inch whole-wheat tortillas

Tomato Tea Salsa (page 196)

2 tablespoons shredded fat-free cheddar cheese

Spray a large nonstick skillet with an olive oil cooking spray. Heat to medium-high. Sauté the peppers for approximately 2 minutes.

Whisk together the egg whites, cilantro, pepper, and dry tea. Add to the pan and scramble until done to your taste.

Heat the tortillas. Remove the eggs from the pan and divide in half placing them in the middle of the tortillas. Top each with 1 tablespoon salsa and ½ tablespoon cheese. Wrap the burritos and serve with the remaining salsa.

Serves 2

NUTRITION PER SERVING (WITH 1 TABLESPOON SALSA): *calories 310, fat 4.5g, protein 26g, carb 41g*

Tomato Tea Salsa

> 4 Roma tomatoes, seeded and chopped (save the seeds to make Tea Tomato-Seed Salad Dressing, page 191)
>
> 1 tablespoon fresh lime juice
>
> Grated zest of ¼ lime
>
> 1 tablespoon your favorite dry tea
>
> 1 jalapeño, seeded and chopped
>
> All-Purpose Fish/Vegetable Tea Rub (page 190) to taste

Combine all the ingredients in a medium bowl.

Serves 2

NUTRITION PER SERVING: *calories 150, fat 4g, protein 25g, carb 3g*

Chocolate Hazelnut Torte Frostea

> Chocolate Hazelnut Torte Rooibos tisane* to cover the bottom of a teapot, or 1 bag chocolate hazelnut–flavored tea
>
> 1 teaspoon agave nectar or any honey, mixed with 1 tablespoon hot water
>
> 1 cup filtered water, boiled
>
> Ice to fill a blender
>
> 1 tablespoon fat- and sugar-free whipped topping (optional)

Combine the tea and agave nectar in a teapot or cup. Add the water and steep for 3 to 4 minutes. Strain the brewed tea mixture over the ice in a blender and blend to your desired thickness. Serve with whipped topping, if desired. Resteep the loose or bagged tea.

*If you do not have the Chocolate Hazelnut Torte Rooibos tisane, use any plain black tea or Rooibos tisane and add ½ teaspoon of mini chocolate chips and a small handful of chopped hazelnuts to the steeping.

Can also be served hot.

Serves 1
NUTRITION PER SERVING: *calories 50, fat 2 g, protein 1 g, carb 7 g*
WITH 1 TABLESPOON SUGAR-FREE WHIPPED TOPPING: *calories 60, fat 2 g, protein 1 g, carb 9 g*

Mediterranean Tea Salad

4 Tea-Grilled Chicken breast halves (page 193)

2 heads romaine lettuce

1 English cucumber, seeded and chopped

8 Kalamata olives, pitted and chopped

1 red bell pepper, seeded and chopped

1 pint cherry tomatoes

½ red onion, chopped

4 ounces crumbled feta cheese (about 1 cup)

2 tablespoons balsamic vinegar

¼ teaspoon Dijon mustard

1 tablespoon olive oil

¼ teaspoon ground black pepper

Pinch of ground dry oolong tea

½ teaspoon chopped cilantro

Chop the chicken into bite-size pieces and place in a large bowl.

Chop the lettuce into bite-size pieces and add to the bowl. Add the cucumber, olives, red pepper, tomatoes, onion, and feta cheese.

In a small bowl, whisk the vinegar and mustard together. Add the olive oil and whisk well. Add the pepper, dry tea and cilantro. Drizzle over the salad and toss together.

Serves 4

NUTRITION PER SERVING: *calories 290, fat 11 g, protein 36 g, carb 15 g*

Lemon Tea Baked Halibut

2 lemons, sliced thin

Four 4-ounce halibut fillets

1 teaspoon olive oil

2 teaspoons All-Purpose Fish/Vegetable Tea Rub (page 190), or add ¼
  teaspoon your favorite finely ground dry tea to any fish seasoning you love

2 anchovy fillets,* rinsed and patted dry

2 teaspoon capers, rinsed and drained

1 teaspoon chopped fresh dill

Heat the oven to 350 degrees F with a rack in the middle. Place half of the lemon slices on the bottom of a baking dish. Place the halibut fillets on the lemon slices. Brush with the olive oil. Rub the fish with the Tea Rub. Chop the anchovies and sprinkle on top of the fish. Cover with the remaining lemon slices. Sprinkle with the capers and dill.

Bake for 20 minutes, or until fish is white and flaky.

*The anchovies will add a depth of flavor and will not taste fishy.

Serves 4

NUTRITION PER SERVING: *calories 150, fat 4 g, protein 25 g, carb 3 g*

Oven-Roasted Tea Asparagus

   1 pound medium-thick asparagus

   2 tablespoons olive oil

   1 teaspoon ground black pepper

   ½ teaspoon kosher salt

   ¼ teaspoon finely ground dry tea you love

   1 tablespoon grated Parmesan cheese (optional)

Heat oven to 375 degrees F.

Bend one asparagus stalk until it snaps. This will tell you where to cut the rest of the asparagus. (The woody part of the stalk is good saved for soup.) Trim all the asparagus.

Place the asparagus on a foil-lined cookie sheet. Drizzle with the olive oil and sprinkle with the pepper, salt, and dry tea. Toss the asparagus to ensure they are evenly seasoned. Bake for approximately 30 minutes. Sprinkle with the cheese, if desired, and roast until cheese is melted.

Serves 4

NUTRITION PER SERVING (WITH CHEESE): *calories 110, fat 7 g, protein 5 g, carb 8 g*

TEAna Colada Frostea

   Green or White Tea with Pineapple* to cover the bottom of the teapot, or 1
      bag pineapple-flavored tea

   1 teaspoon agave nectar or any honey, mixed with 1 tablespoon hot water

   2 tablespoons Torani Sugar-Free Coconut syrup, or any sugar-free coconut
      syrup

   1 cup filtered water, boiled

   Ice to fill a blender

   I tablespoon fat- and sugar-free whipped topping (optional)

Combine the tea, agave nectar, and syrup in the teapot or cup. Add the water and steep for 3 minutes. Strain the brewed tea mixture over the ice in a blender and blend to your desired thickness. Serve with whipped topping, if desired. Resteep the loose or bagged tea.

*If you do not have a tea with pineapple, use any plain White or Green Tea or Rooibos tisane and add 1 tablespoon chopped dried or fresh pineapple while steeping.

Can also be served hot.

Serves 1

NUTRITION PER SERVING: *calories 50, fat 0g, protein 1g, carb 12g*

WITH 1 TABLESPOON SUGAR-FREE WHIPPED TOPPING: *calories 60, fat 0g, protein 1g,*
   carb 14

DAY 3

Blueberry Pie Frostea

> *White Blueberry Tea* to cover the bottom of a teapot or 1 bag blueberry-*
>   *flavored tea*
> *1 teaspoon agave nectar or any honey, mixed with 1 tablespoon hot water*
> *1 cup filtered water, boiled*
> *Ice to fill a blender*

Combine the tea and agave nectar in a teapot or cup. Add the water and steep for 3 minutes. Strain the brewed tea mixture over the ice in a blender and blend to your desired thickness. Serve. Resteep the loose or bagged tea.

*If you do not have a blueberry tea, use any plain white or green tea or Rooibos tisane and add 1 tablespoon fresh or dried blueberries while steeping.

Can also be served hot.

Serves 1

NUTRITION PER SERVING: *calories 60, fat 0g, protein 1g, carb 14g*

Vegetable Tea Soup with Chicken

Four 4-ounce skinless, boneless chicken breast halves

2 teaspoons olive oil

½ cup chopped onion

2 cloves garlic, chopped fine

2 cups shredded cabbage

2 cups low-sodium chicken or vegetable broth

½ cup chopped carrots

½ cup chopped celery

One 14.5-ounce can chopped tomatoes

½ cup chopped green beans

½ cup chopped zucchini

1 teaspoon ground black pepper

1 tablespoon finely ground dry oolong tea

2 tablespoons Worcestershire sauce

1 tablespoon chopped fresh basil or 1 teaspoon dry

2 tablespoons grated fat-free Parmesan cheese

Heat the olive oil in a medium saucepan over medium heat. Add the onion and cook until translucent. Add the garlic and stir, being careful not to burn it. Add the cabbage and sauté for about 10 minutes. Add the broth and 1½ cups water.

Add the carrots, celery, and tomatoes with their juice. Cook for 30 minutes.

Add the green beans, zucchini, pepper, dry tea, Worcestershire sauce, and basil. Cook for 15 minutes more. Add the Parmesan cheese before serving.

This recipe may be doubled and kept in refrigerator or freezer.

Serves 4

NUTRITION PER SERVING: *calories 240, fat 4.5 g, protein 33 g, carb 16 g*

Turkey Tea Meatloaf

½ cup brewed oolong tea

¾ cup quick-cooking oats

1 tablespoon olive oil

1 small onion, chopped

½ cup chopped red or orange bell peppers

2 cups loosely packed fresh spinach leaves, chopped

2 pounds ground turkey breast

4 egg whites, beaten

¼ cup ketchup

1 tablespoon Worcestershire sauce

1 teaspoon ground black pepper

Olive oil cooking spray

1 8-ounce can tomato sauce

Heat the oven to 350 degrees F. Pour the brewed tea over the oats and set aside.

Heat the olive oil in a medium sauté pan. Cook the onion over medium heat for a few minutes, until translucent.

Add the bell peppers and cook for approximately 1 minute. Add the spinach, stir, and allow to wilt. Remove the pan from the heat and allow to cool.

Mix the turkey, egg whites, oats, ketchup, 2 teaspoons of the Worcestershire sauce, the pepper, oats and the cooled vegetables.

Spray the bottom of a 13- by 9-inch baking dish with olive oil cooking spray. Form the turkey into a loaf approximately 5 inches wide and 8 inches long. Mix the tomato sauce and remaining 1 teaspoon Worcestershire sauce and pour over the meatloaf.

Bake for approximately 1 hour, until the internal temperature measures 160 degrees F. Allow to rest for 10 minutes before slicing.

Serves 8

NUTRITION PER SERVING: *calories 200, fat 4 g, protein 32 g, carb 12 g*

Baked Tea Pears

2 pears, peeled, halved, and cored

½ cup brewed fruit tea, any flavor

2 packets dry stevia

½ teaspoon ground cinnamon

Heat the oven to 350 degrees F.

Place the pears in a baking dish. Pour the brewed tea over the pears. Sprinkle with the stevia and cinnamon. Bake for 40 to 50 minutes until fork tender, spooning the tea over the pears halfway through the cooking process.

Allow pears to cool to room temperature before serving.

Serves 4

NUTRITION PER SERVING: *calories 50, fat 0g, protein 0g, carb 12g*

Strawberry-Balsamic Tea Sauce

1 cup strawberries

2 tablespoons balsamic vinegar

2 tablespoons your favorite brewed tea

Pinch of ground black pepper

1 teaspoon brown sugar

Chop the berries into small pieces. Combine with the vinegar, brewed tea, pepper, and sugar in a small saucepan. Stir well. Cook on a low heat for approximately 10 minutes, until the strawberries are soft.

This sauce can also be made without cooking. Simply combine all the ingredients in a bowl and allow to macerate for at least 30 minutes. The sauce will be thinner and the strawberries chunky, but equally delicious.

Serves 4

NUTRITION PER SERVING: *calories 20, fat 0g, protein 0g, carb 5g*

DAY 4

Vegetable Mushroom Tea Frittata

½ pound mushrooms (any kind you love), cleaned and diced

2 green onions (scallions), trimmed and sliced

½ cup diced green, red, or yellow bell pepper

2 pinches of any dry tea you love

1 stalk celery, chopped

1 cup brewed tea (any kind you love)

Pinch of cayenne pepper (optional)

8 egg whites

Heat a large nonstick skillet. Add the mushrooms, green onions, bell peppers, dry tea, and celery.

Add the brewed tea to the skillet, cover, and bring to a simmer. If you want it a little spicy, add a pinch of cayenne pepper. Stir occasionally. Cook until vegetables are done to your taste.

Beat egg whites in bowl. When vegetables are done, pour in egg mixture. Cover and cook over a low heat until firm.

Serves 2

NUTRITION PER SERVING: *calories 140, fat 0.5 g, protein 23 g, carb 10 g*

Ginger Bread Hot Todtea

Ginger Bread Rooibos tisane* to cover the bottom of a teapot or 1 bag
   ginger-flavored tea

1 cup filtered water, boiled

1 teaspoon agave nectar or any honey, mixed with 1 tablespoon hot water

1 tablespoon fat- and sugar-free whipped topping (optional)

Combine the tea and agave nectar in a teapot or cup. Add the water and steep for 4 minutes. Serve hot with whipped topping, if desired.

*If you do not have the Ginger Bread Rooibos, use any plain tea or Rooibos tisane and add ½ teaspoon dried ginger, 1 tablespoon grated orange zest, ½ teaspoon chopped almonds, and 3 whole pink peppercorns to the steeping.

If you desire a Frostea, strain the brewed tea mixture over ice in a blender and blend to your desired thickness. Serve with whipped topping, if desired. Resteep the loose or bagged tea.

Serves 1
NUTRITION PER SERVING: *calories 50, fat 1.5g, protein 1g, carb 9g*
WITH 1 TABLESPOON WHIPPED TOPPING: *calories 60, fat 1.5g, protein 1g, carb 10g*

Tea Chicken Tostadas with Tomato Tea Salsa

Four 8-inch whole-wheat tortillas

1 teaspoon olive oil

1 pound skinless, boneless chicken breast halves

½ teaspoon ground black pepper

¼ teaspoon finely ground dry oolong tea

4 to 5 drops of hot sauce, such as Tabasco

2 heads romaine lettuce

4 tomatoes, chopped

½ cup grated carrots

1 medium avocado

1 large cucumber, peeled, seeded, and chopped

1 red onion, chopped

¼ cup chopped cilantro

Juice of 2 limes

1 jalapeño, seeded and chopped (optional)

¼ cup shredded fat-free Cheddar cheese

Tomato Tea Salsa (page 196)

Heat the oven to 450 degrees F. Brush tortillas with olive oil and toast in the oven until crispy.

Season the chicken with the pepper, dry tea, and hot sauce. Grill in a hot grill pan until browned on both sides, approximately 8 minutes. Set aside to cool, then chop into bite-size pieces.

Slice the romaine in half lengthwise. Place on the grill pan for 1 to 2 minutes, to wilt slightly. Remove from the pan and chop very coarsely.

Put the lettuce, tomatoes, and carrots in a large bowl. Add the chicken.

Cut the avocados in half and remove the pits. Scoop out the flesh. Chop the avocados into cubes and place in a medium bowl. Add the cucumber, onion, cilantro and lime juice. If you like, add the jalapeño to the bowl.

Place the tortillas onto 4 plates. Divide the salad among the 4 plates. Top with the avocado mixture. Sprinkle each salad with 1 tablespoon Cheddar cheese. Serve the salsa on the side.

Serves 8
NUTRITION PER SERVING (WITHOUT SALSA): *calories 230, fat 6 g, protein 20 g, carb 32 g*

Mint Chocolate Ice Cream Frostea

Any mint chocolate tea or Rooibos tisane* to cover the bottom of a teapot or
  1 bag mint chocolate–flavored tea
1 teaspoon agave nectar, or any honey, mixed with 1 tablespoon hot water
1 cup filtered water, boiled
Ice to fill a blender

Combine the tea and agave nectar in a teapot or cup. Add the water and steep for 3 minutes. Strain the brewed tea mixture over the ice in a blender and blend to your desired thickness. Serve. Resteep the loose or bagged tea.

*If you do not have a mint chocolate tea or Rooibos tisane, use any plain white or green tea or Rooibos tisane and add 1 teaspoon chopped fresh or dried mint and 1 teaspoon mini chocolate chips while steeping.

Can also be served hot.

Serves 1

NUTRITION PER SERVING: *calories 50, fat 1.5 g, protein 1 g, carb 9 g*

DAY 5

Apple-Cinnamon Tea Oatmeal

> Oatmeal for 1 serving
> 3 pinches of ground dry tea, any kind you love
> 1 tablespoon chopped almonds
> ¼ cup chopped apples
> Ground cinnamon

Prepare the oatmeal as per package instructions. Add the dry tea to the oatmeal. Top with the almonds and apples. Dust with cinnamon.

Serves 1

NUTRITION PER SERVING: *calories 210, fat 6 g, protein 8 g, carb 31 g*

Strawberry-Raspberry Pie DaiquirTEA Frostea

> Any strawberry- or raspberry-flavored tea or tisane* to cover the bottom of a
>   tea pot or 1 bag strawberry- or raspberry-flavored tea
> 1 teaspoon agave nectar or any honey, mixed with 1 tablespoon
>   hot water
> 1 cup filtered water, boiled
> Ice to fill a blender
> 1 tablespoon fat- and sugar-free whipped topping (optional)

Combine the tea and agave nectar in a teapot or cup. Add the water and steep for 4 minutes. Strain the brewed tea mixture over the ice in a blender and blend to your desired thickness. Serve with whipped topping, if desired. Resteep the loose or bagged tea.

*If you do not have a strawberry- or raspberry-flavored tea or Rooibos tisane, use any plain Tea or Rooibos tisane and add 1 tablespoon chopped fresh or dried strawberries or raspberries to the steeping.

Can also be served hot.

Serves 1
NUTRITION PER SERVING: *calories 45, fat 0g, protein 1g, carb 10g*
WITH 1 TABLESPOON WHIPPED TOPPING: *calories 50, Fat 0g, protein 1g, carb 12g*

Tea Garden Grilled Salmon

> *Four 4-ounce salmon fillets or one 16-ounce fillet*
> *Olive oil cooking spray*
> *2 teaspoons All-Purpose Fish/Vegetable Tea Rub (page 190) or add ⅓*
> *teaspoon any finely ground dry tea to your favorite fish seasoning*
> *Olive oil*

Rinse and pat the salmon dry. Spray the olive oil on both sides of the salmon. Rub the seasoning on both sides of the salmon.

Heat a grill pan or barbeque to high.

Using a small amount of olive oil on a paper towel, rub the grill pan or barbeque grill to prevent the fish from sticking.

Grill the salmon for 5 minutes on each side. Remove from the grill, cover with foil, and allow to rest for 5 minutes before serving.

This fish may be served hot, at room temperature, or chilled on a salad.

Serves 4
NUTRITION PER SERVING: *calories 189, fat 8g, protein 26g, carb 1g*

BBQ Tea–Grilled Chicken

> *Four 6-ounce skinless, boneless chicken breast halves*
>
> *1 tablespoon olive oil*
>
> *1 tablespoon balsamic vinegar*
>
> *2 teaspoons Chicken Tea Rub (page 189) or BBQ Tea Rub (page 190), add*
>
> > *¼ teaspoon finely ground dry tea to your best chicken seasoning*

Wash and pat dry the chicken breasts. Mix the oil and vinegar and rub into the chicken. Sprinkle lightly with the chicken seasoning. Allow to sit for 10 minutes.

Heat a grill pan or barbeque to high. Grill the chicken until well browned, about 8 minutes.

Serves 4

NUTRITION PER SERVING: *calories 170, fat 3 g, protein 28 g, carb 5 g*

Tiramisu Rooibos Hot Todtea Tisane

> *Tiramisu Rooibos tisane* to cover the bottom of a teapot or 1 bag plain black*
> > *tea or Rooibos tisane*
>
> *1 teaspoon agave nectar or any honey, mixed with 1 tablespoon hot water*
>
> *1 cup filtered water, boiled*
>
> *1 tablespoon fat- and sugar-free whipped topping (optional)*

Combine the tea and agave nectar in a teapot or cup. Add the water and steep for 3 to 4 minutes and serve hot with whipped topping, if desired.

*If you do not have the Tiramisu Rooibos tisane, use any plain Black Tea or Rooibos tisane and add ½ teaspoon mini chocolate chips, ½ teaspoon chopped almonds, and ¼ teaspoon almond extract to the steeping.

If you desire a Frostea, strain the brewed tea mixture over ice in a blender and blend to your desired thickness. Serve with whipped topping, if desired. Resteep the loose or bagged tea.

Serves 1

NUTRITION PER SERVING: *calories 50, fat 2g, protein 1g, carb 8g*

WITH 1 TABLESPOON WHIPPED TOPPING: *calories 60, fat 2g, protein 1g, carb 9g*

DAY 6

Tea Popsicles

Any Frostea you love (double recipe)

6 unit Popsicle tray and sticks

Prepare Frostea, doubling the recipe. Let the ice melt for 20 to 30 minutes. Pour the mixture into the Popsicle trays, insert the sticks, and place in the freezer. Freeze until firm, 1 hour or more.

Serves 6

NUTRITION PER SERVING: *Varies according to Frostea recipe used*

Tea Chicken Stir-Fry

2 tablespoons olive oil

½ teaspoon red pepper flakes

1 teaspoon chopped fresh thyme or ½ teaspoon dried

1 pound skinless, boneless chicken breasts, sliced into strips

1 red onion, sliced

1 pound crimini mushrooms, sliced

1 red bell pepper, sliced

1 green bell pepper, sliced

2 cups chopped broccoli florets

½ cup brewed oolong tea

Juice 2 lemons

½ teaspoon ground black pepper

1 cup snow peas

Grated zest of 1 lemon

Tea Rice (page 193), for serving

Heat the olive oil over medium-high heat in a large skillet or wok. Add the red pepper flakes and thyme. Cook for just a few seconds to allow the seasoning to infuse into the oil.

Add the chicken. Cook for 3 minutes, stirring constantly, and remove from the pan.

Add the onion to the pan. Cook until translucent. Add the mushrooms and cook for a few minutes longer. Add the red and green bell peppers and the broccoli. Cook for a few minutes.

Add the chicken back into the pan. Add the tea, lemon juice, and pepper. Add the snow peas. Add the lemon zest and cook for just a few minutes more. Serve with Tea Rice.

Serves 4

NUTRITION PER SERVING (WITHOUT RICE): *calories 240, fat 5 g, protein 33 g, carb 18 g*

Orange Sherbet Frostea

Any orange-vanilla green or white tea* to cover the bottom of a teapot or

 1 bag orange-vanilla–flavored tea

1 teaspoon agave nectar or any honey, mixed with 1 tablespoon hot water

1 cup filtered water, boiled

Ice to fill a blender

Combine the tea and agave nectar in a teapot or cup. Add the water and steep for 3 minutes. Strain the brewed tea mixture over the ice in a blender and blend to your desired thickness. Serve. Resteep the loose or bagged tea.

*If you do not have an orange-vanilla tea, use any plain white or green tea, or Rooibos tisane and add 1 tablespoon chopped fresh or dried orange peel and ½ teaspoon vanilla extract while steeping.

Can also be served hot.

Serves 1

NUTRITION PER SERVING: *calories 35, fat 0 g, protein 1 g, carb 8 g*

DAY 7

Fruit Tea Smoothie

> *1 cup frozen blueberries or strawberries*
> *½ cup your favorite brewed fruit or vanilla tea*
> *1½ cups plain nonfat yogurt*
> *1 teaspoon honey*

Place all ingredients in a blender and blend until smooth and frothy.

Serves 1

NUTRITION PER SERVING: *calories 270, fat 5 g, protein 17 g, carb 49 g*

Caramel-Banana DaiquirTEA Frostea

> *Any caramel black tea or Rooibos tisane* to cover the bottom of a teapot or 1*
> *bag caramel-flavored tea*
> *1 teaspoon agave nectar or any honey, mixed with 1 tablespoon*
> *hot water*
> *1 or 2 tablespoons diced fresh bananas*
> *1 cup filtered water, boiled*
> *Ice to fill a blender*

Combine the tea and agave nectar in a teapot or cup. Add the water and steep for 3 minutes. Strain the brewed tea mixture over the ice in a blender and blend to your desired thickness. Serve. Resteep the loose or bagged tea.

*If you do not have a caramel-flavored tea or Rooibos tisane, use any plain black tea or Rooibos and add 1 teaspoon caramel bits to the steep.

Can also be served hot.

Serves 1

NUTRITION PER SERVING: *calories 60, fat 0 g, protein 1 g, carb 14 g*

Tea Orange Turkey Breast

> *Juice of 1 orange*
>
> *8 turkey breast cutlets*
>
> *1 tablespoon all-purpose flour*
>
> *¼ teaspoon finely ground dry oolong tea*
>
> *¼ teaspoon kosher salt*
>
> *1 teaspoon ground black pepper*
>
> *¼ teaspoon ground ginger*
>
> *2 tablespoons olive oil*

Pour half of the orange juice over the turkey cutlets and allow to sit in the refrigerator for 30 minutes. Put the flour, dry tea, salt, pepper, and ginger in a large resealable plastic bag. Add the turkey and shake until evenly coated.

Heat the olive oil in a large skillet. Add the turkey and cook on both sides until browned, approximately 12 minutes. Drizzle with the remaining orange juice.

Serves 8

NUTRITION PER SERVING: *calories 200, fat 8 g, protein 28 g, carb 5 g*

Tea Chicken Pasta with Artichokes and Sun-Dried Tomatoes

> *Olive oil cooking spray*
>
> *2 tablespoons olive oil*
>
> *1 medium red onion, sliced*
>
> *1 pound skinless, boneless chicken breast halves*
>
> *1 teaspoon Chicken Tea Rub (page 189) or any poultry rub you love plus ¼*
> *teaspoon finely ground tea*
>
> *½ teaspoon dried oregano*

1 lemon, halved crosswise

One 14-ounce can artichoke hearts, drained and quartered

1 tablespoon chopped sun-dried tomatoes (oil packed, drained)

1 teaspoon dry oolong tea or any other dry tea

8 ounces whole-wheat pasta

Heat the oven to 350 degrees F.

Spray a large baking dish with olive oil cooking spray and set aside.

On medium-high heat, heat the olive oil in a large nonstick skillet. Add the onion and cook until softened. Place in the bottom of the baking dish.

Season the chicken with the Tea Rub, oregano, and juice of half of the lemon. Cook in the skillet until brown on both sides. Layer the chicken on top of the onions in the baking dish.

Slice the remaining half of the lemon into very thin slices and place over the chicken, along with the artichokes and sun-dried tomatoes. Bake uncovered for approximately 20 minutes.

Meanwhile, bring a large pot of water to a boil. Reduce the heat to a low simmer. Add the oolong tea and allow to steep for 3 minutes. Strain the tea leaves from the water and bring back to a boil. (You can resteep the leaves while you cook.) Add the pasta and cook according to package directions. Drain the pasta. Serve the chicken and vegetables over the pasta.

Serves 4

NUTRITION PER SERVING: *calories 310, fat 6g, protein 26g, carb 39g*

Tea-Poached Apricots or Plums

2 quarts filtered water

4 tablespoons your favorite dry black tea

1 cup rice wine vinegar

1 teaspoon ground cinnamon

    1 teaspoon ground cloves (optional)

    2 tablespoons vanilla extract

    4 pounds fresh apricots or your favorite plums

    Tea Custard Sauce (page 215, optional)

Bring the filtered water to a boil and set aside for a few minutes. Add the tea and steep for 3 minutes. Strain into a large stainless-steel saucepan. (Resteep the tea during your cooking, if you like.)

Add the vinegar, cinnamon, cloves (if using), and vanilla to the tea. Add the fruit and simmer over low heat for about 10 minutes. Set aside to cool. Remove the fruit and take off the skins. Cut in half and remove the pits. Place the fruit back into the pan, cover, and refrigerate until cold.

Serve with Tea Custard Sauce, if you like. Two whole fruits (4 halves) makes a meal and one whole fruit (two halves) makes a dessert. The tea-poached fruit could also be used as a side dish to any meal, or as a topping on nonfat cottage cheese or yogurt.

Serves 4

NUTRITION PER SERVING 2 WHOLE FRUITS (WITHOUT SAUCE): *calories 280, fat 4.5 g, protein 3 g, carb 46 g*

Tea Custard Sauce

    ⅓ cup nonfat evaporated milk

    2 tablespoons brewed vanilla tea or tisane or any brewed tea or tisane you love

    1 egg

    2 teaspoons sugar

    ¼ teaspoon vanilla extract

Heat the milk and brewed tea in a small saucepan until tiny bubbles form around the edges.

In a heatproof bowl that will fit over a medium saucepan, beat the egg and sugar until sugar is totally dissolved. Add the hot milk and tea gradually, beating continuously so that the egg does not curdle.

Place the bowl over a medium saucepan of hot water (not boiling). Stir in the vanilla. Cook, stirring continuously with a wooden spoon, until thick enough to coat the back of the spoon.

Remove from the heat. Cover the sauce with plastic wrap, with the wrap touching the top of the custard. This will prevent the sauce from forming a skin on the top. May be served warm or chilled over poached apricots or plums, or over any fresh fruit or dessert you like.

Serves 4
NUTRITION PER SERVING: *calories 35, fat 1 g, protein 2 g, carb 3 g*

DAY 8

Egg White Tea Scramble

Green tea
1 tablespoon olive oil
½ cup sliced crimini or button mushrooms
½ cup chopped bell pepper, any color
1 cup loosely packed baby spinach
12 egg whites
¼ teaspoon ground black pepper
Pinch of red pepper flakes
2 tablespoons grated fat-free Parmesan cheese

Brew some green tea and set 2 tablespoons aside to cool. Enjoy the rest of the tea while preparing your scramble.

Heat the olive oil in a large nonstick skillet. Add the mushrooms and cook until softened. If the oil is totally absorbed you can add a little brewed green tea to the pan. Add the bell peppers and cook for a few minutes. Add the spinach and cook until wilted.

In a small bowl, lightly whisk the egg whites, 2 tablespoons brewed tea, black pepper and red pepper flakes. Add the egg mixture to the pan and cook, stirring, until done to your taste. Add the cheese just before serving.

Serves 4

NUTRITION PER SERVING: *calories 130, fat 4 g, protein 17 g, carb 7 g*

Caramel Apple Hot Todtea

Caramel Rooibos tisane* to cover the bottom of a teapot or 1 bag caramel-flavored tea

1 teaspoon agave nectar or any honey, mixed with 1 tablespoon hot water

1 tablespoon peeled and cubed fresh or dried apple

1 cup filtered water, boiled

Combine the tea, agave nectar, and apples in a teapot or cup. Add the water and steep for 3 to 4 minutes, strain, and serve hot.

*If you do not have Caramel Rooibos use any plain black tea or Rooibos tisane and add 1 teaspoon of caramel bits to the steeping.

If you desire a Frostea, strain the brewed tea mixture over ice in a blender and blend to your desired thickness. Serve. Resteep the loose or bagged tea.

Serves 1

NUTRITION PER SERVING: *calories 60, fat 0 g, protein 1 g, carb 14 g*

Cold Chicken or Turkey Tea Salad

Four pieces Tea-Grilled Chicken (page 193), BBQ Tea–Grilled Chicken (page 209), Tea Orange Turkey Breast (page 213), or Rosemary Orange Tea Chicken (page 225)

1 orange or blood orange

½ grapefruit

1 bulb fennel, sliced thin

2 heads romaine lettuce, chopped

One 16-ounce package shredded cabbage and carrots (cole slaw mix)

2 tablespoons slivered almonds

¼ teaspoon ground black pepper

⅛ teaspoon finely ground dry oolong tea

½ teaspoon Dijon mustard

2 tablespoons olive oil

Slice the chicken into bite-size pieces and place into a large salad bowl.

Grate the zest from the orange and set aside. Cut the orange in half horizontally. Squeeze the juice from one half and set aside. Cut off and discard the outside membrane from the other half and separate the sections. Cut the sections into chunks.

Cut off and discard the peel and membrane from the grapefruit. Separate the sections and cut into large chunks.

Add the chicken, orange and grapefruit chunks, fennel, romaine, cabbage mix, and almonds.

In a small bowl, whisk together the orange zest and juice, pepper, dry tea, and mustard. Add the olive oil. Whisk together and drizzle over the salad. Toss to mix.

Serves 4

NUTRITION PER SERVING: *calories 400, fat 11 g, protein 32 g, carb 49 g*

Cauliflower Tea Mash

1 teaspoon dry oolong tea

2 cups boiling water

1 clove garlic

1 pound cauliflower florets, preferably fresh but frozen are okay

½ cup low-sodium chicken broth

2 tablespoons grated fat-free Parmesan cheese (optional)

Salt

Ground black pepper

Brew the tea for 10 minutes in the water. Strain the tea into a large saucepan. (Resteep the tea leaves for a cup of tea while you cook.)

Add the garlic to the saucepan. Add the cauliflower. Add water to cover the cauliflower. Bring to a boil. Reduce the heat to medium. Simmer until fork-tender (approximately 12 minutes). Save 2 tablespoons of the liquid; drain the rest.

Transfer the cauliflower, garlic, and reserved liquid to the bowl of a food processor. Add the chicken broth slowly while processing until cauliflower is smooth. Add the Parmesan cheese, if you like. Season to taste with salt and pepper.

Serves 4

NUTRITION PER SERVING (WITH CHEESE): *calories 60, fat .5 g, protein 6 g, carb 9 g*

Tea Fruit Salad

> *½ cup any brewed fruit tea*
> *Juice of 1 lemon*
> *2 teaspoons honey*
> *1 teaspoon chopped fresh mint*
> *1 pound strawberries*
> *1 pound blueberries*
> *1 pound raspberries*
> *3 kiwis, peeled and sliced*

During winter months when berries are unavailable they can be substituted with winter fruit or frozen sugar-free.

Combine the brewed tea, lemon juice, honey, and mint. Put all the fruit in a large bowl. Pour the topping over the fruit before serving.

Serves 4

NUTRITION PER SERVING: *calories 130, fat 0 g, protein 2 g, carb 36 g*

CappuTEAno Frostea

> Roasted Oolong Tea to cover ½ of the teapot (or any oolong or black tea) or
> 1 bag oolong tea
> 1 teaspoon agave nectar or any honey, mixed with 1 tablespoon of hot water
> 1 tablespoon Torani Sugar-Free Coffee Syrup, or any sugar-free coffee syrup
> 1½ teaspoons any Torani Sugar-Free Hazelnut Syrup, or any sugar-free
> hazelnut syrup
> 1 cup filtered water, boiled
> Ice to fill a blender
> 1 tablespoon fat- and sugar-free whipped topping (optional)

Combine the tea, agave nectar, and syrups in a teapot or cup. Add the water and steep for 5 minutes. Strain the brewed tea mixture over the ice in a blender and blend to your desired thickness. Serve with whipped topping, if desired. Resteep the loose or bagged tea.

Can also be served hot.

Serves 1
NUTRITION PER SERVING: *calories: 25, fat 0 g, protein 1 g, carb 6 g*
WITH 1 TABLESPOON WHIPPED TOPPING: *calories 30, fat, 0 g, protein 1 g, carb 7 g*

DAY 9

Cinnamon Roast Hot Todtea

> Cinnamon Roast Rooibos tisane* to cover the bottom of a teapot or 1 bag
> cinnamon-flavored tea
> 1 teaspoon agave nectar or any honey, mixed with 1 tablespoon hot water
> 1 cup filtered water, boiled
> 1 tablespoon fat- and sugar-free whipped topping (optional)

Combine the tea and agave nectar in a teapot or cup. Steep for 3 to 4 minutes, strain, and serve hot with whipped topping, if desired.

*If you do not have Cinnamon Roast Rooibos, use any plain black tea or Rooibos tisane and add ½ teaspoon ground cinnamon to the steeping.

If you desire a Frostea, strain the brewed tea mixture over ice in a blender and blend to your desired thickness. Serve with whipped topping, if desired. Resteep the loose or bagged tea.

Serves 1
NUTRITION PER SERVING: *calories 30, fat 0 g, protein 1 g, carb 7 g*
WITH 1 TABLESPOON WHIPPED TOPPING: *calories 35, Fat 0 g, protein 1 g, carb 8 g*

Tea Salad Niçoise

8 small red potatoes (about ½ pound)

1 tablespoon any dry Tea you love

1 pound green beans, trimmed

1 pound fresh tuna fillet, cut in 6 pieces

Olive oil cooking spray

¼ teaspoon All-Purpose Fish/Vegetable Tea Rub (page 190) or any season-ings you love mixed with a pinch of any finely ground dry tea you love

One 5- to 7-ounce Spring Mix Salad Mix

1 pint cherry tomatoes

1 small bunch radishes, trimmed and sliced (optional)

2 tablespoons capers, rinsed and drained

16 pitted Kalamata olives

4 anchovy fillets (optional)

2 tablespoons olive oil

¼ cup balsamic vinegar

Fill a large bowl with ice and water.

In a small saucepan, boil the potatoes with the dry tea in water to cover until fork tender. Remove the potatoes from the boiling water and set aside to cool. Keep the tea water. Slice the potatoes when cool enough to handle and set aside.

Cook the green beans for 5 minutes in the same boiling tea water used for the potatoes. Remove with a slotted spoon and immediately place in the ice water to bring the beans to room temperature quickly. Remove the beans from the ice water, clean off any tea leaves (or keep them as I do) and set aside.

Heat a grill pan to hot. Spray the tuna on both sides with olive oil cooking spray. Sprinkle lightly with All-Purpose Fish/Vegetable Tea Rub. Grill on the grill pan; the tuna may be just seared or cooked through, as you prefer. Set aside.

On a large platter, use the lettuce mix for a bed for the other vegetables and fish. Top with the tomatoes, sliced radishes (if using), green beans, potatoes, capers, and olives. Halve the anchovy fillets and add them to the salad, if you like. Place the tuna on top.

Mix the olive oil and balsamic vinegar. Drizzle over the top and serve.

Serves 6
NUTRITION PER SERVING: *calories 410, fat 13 g, protein 27 g, carb 50 g*

Baked Tea Apples

> *4 medium apples*
>
> *1 cup brewed Caramel Dream Tea or any sweet tea you love*
>
> *4 packages stevia, sugar substitute, or any other noncaloric sweetener you love*
>
> *1 teaspoon ground cinnamon*
>
> *2 tablespoons chopped walnuts*
>
> *2 tablespoons raisins or currants*
>
> *1 tablespoon honey*

Preheat the oven to 350 degrees F.

Cut the tops off the apples and set aside. Remove the cores, being careful not to cut through the bottom of the apples. Place the apples in a shallow baking dish. Pour the tea over the apples. Sprinkle half of the stevia and the cinnamon on the apples. Push the walnuts and raisins into the apple cavities.

Place the tops on the apples. Drizzle with the honey. Sprinkle the remaining cinnamon and stevia over the tops. Bake for 45 minutes or until fork tender.

Delicious eaten warm.

Serves 4
NUTRITION PER SERVING: *calories 120, fat 2.5 g, protein 1 g, carb 28 g*

Grilled Tea Steak

> *1 pound beef tenderloin, trimmed and cut into 4 portions*
> *Olive oil cooking spray*
> *3 teaspoons Steak Tea Rub (page 190) or ¼ teaspoon finely ground dry Tea*
>   *added to your favorite steak seasonings*

Allow the steaks to rest out of the refrigerator for 30 minutes to come to room temperature. Meanwhile, heat a grill pan or barbecue to medium-hot. Spray both sides of the steaks with olive oil cooking spray. Rub the Steak Rub into the steaks on both sides. Grill on a barbeque or grill pan to your desired doneness. Remove from the heat. Cover loosely and allow to rest for 10 minutes before serving.

Serves 4
NUTRITION PER SERVING: *calories 120, fat 11 g, protein 22 g, carb 0 g*

Dr. Tea's Candy Bar Black Tea Hot Todtea

> *Dr. Tea's Candy Bar Black Tea* to cover the bottom of a tea pot or 1 bag plain*
>   *Black Tea*
> *1 teaspoon agave nectar or any honey, mixed with 1 tablespoon hot water*
> *1 cup filtered water, boiled*

Combine the tea and agave nectar in a teapot or cup. Add the water and steep for 4 minutes. Strain and serve hot.

*If you do not have the Candy Bar Tea, use any plain Tea or Rooibos tisane and add ½ teaspoon mini chocolate chips and ½ teaspoon caramel bits to the steeping.

If you desire a Frostea, strain the brewed tea mixture over ice in a blender and blend to your desired thickness. Serve. Resteep the loose or bagged tea.

Serves 1

NUTRITION PER SERVING: *calories 45, fat 1g, protein 1g, carb 9g*

D A Y   1 0

Goat Cheese Tea Egg Scramble

1 teaspoon olive oil

4 pieces sun-dried tomatoes, drained if oil-packed, chopped fine

1 cup loosely packed baby spinach

6 egg whites

2 tablespoons nonfat milk

¼ teaspoon ground black pepper

⅛ teaspoon finely ground dry green tea

2 ounces soft goat cheese (about ½ cup), crumbled

Heat the olive oil in a large nonstick skillet over medium heat. Add the tomatoes and cook for just a few minutes. Add the spinach and cook until the spinach wilts.

Whisk together the egg whites, milk, pepper, and dry tea. Add the egg mixture to the pan.

Add the goat cheese when the eggs are almost done. Stir until the eggs are cooked through.

Serves 2

NUTRITION PER SERVING: *calories 160, fat 6g, protein 20g, carb 6g*

Chocolate Cream Pie Hot Todtea

> Chocolate Cream Pie Black Tea* to cover the bottom of a teapot or 1 bag
> chocolate-flavored tea
>
> 1 teaspoon agave nectar or any honey, mixed with 1 tablespoon hot water
>
> 1 cup filtered water, boiled
>
> 1 tablespoon fat- and sugar-free whipped topping (optional)

Combine the tea and agave nectar in a teapot or cup. Add the water and steep for 4 minutes and serve hot with whipped topping, if desired.

*If you do not have the Chocolate Cream Pie Tea, use any plain tea or Rooibos tisane and add ½ teaspoon mini chocolate chips to the steeping.

If you desire a Frostea, strain the brewed tea mixture over ice in a blender and blend to your desired thickness. Serve with whipped topping, if desired. Resteep the loose or bagged tea.

Serves 1

NUTRITION PER SERVING: *calories 35, fat 0.5 g, protein 1 g, carb 7 g*

WITH 1 TABLESPOON WHIPPED TOPPING: *calories 45, fat 0.5 g, protein 1 g, carb 9 g*

Rosemary Orange Tea Chicken

> ¼ cup olive oil
>
> 2 oranges
>
> 1 teaspoon ground black pepper
>
> ½ teaspoon kosher salt
>
> 2 teaspoons chopped fresh rosemary or 1 teaspoon of dried, plus fresh sprigs
> for garnish
>
> ¼ teaspoon finely ground green tea
>
> 1½ pounds skinless, boneless chicken breast halves

Mix together the olive oil, juice of 1½ oranges (set aside the other half), pepper, salt, chopped rosemary, and dry tea. Pour this marinade into a large resealable plastic bag. Add the chicken, seal the bag and refrigerate for at least 30 minutes.

Heat a grill pan or barbecue until hot. Remove chicken from the bag, discarding the remaining marinade, and grill until browned on both sides. Thinly slice the remaining orange half and serve with the chicken. Decorate with a sprig of rosemary.

Serves 4
NUTRITION PER SERVING: *calories 170, fat 2.5 g, protein 28 g, carb 8 g*

DAY 11

Tea-Infused Oatmeal

Oatmeal for 1 serving
3 pinches of your favorite finely ground dry tea

Prepare the oatmeal per package instructions, adding the tea during cooking.

Serves 1
NUTRITION PER SERVING: *calories 150, fat 2.5 g, protein 6 g, carb 25 g*

Vanilla Berry Blast Frostea

Vanilla Berry Rooibos tisane* to cover the bottom of a teapot or 1 bag vanilla-
   flavored tea
1 teaspoon agave nectar or any honey, mixed with 1 tablespoon hot water
1 cup filtered water, boiled
Ice to fill a blender

Combine the tea and agave nectar in a teapot or cup. Add the water and steep for 4 minutes. Strain the brewed tea mixture over the ice in a blender and blend to your desired thickness. Serve. Resteep the loose or bagged tea.

*If you do not have a Vanilla Berry Tea or tisane use any plain tea or Rooibos tisane and add 1 tablespoon fresh or dried berries of your choice and ¼ teaspoon vanilla extract to the steeping.

Can also be served hot.

Serves 1

NUTRITION PER SERVING: *calories 50, fat 0g, protein 1g, carb 10g*

Chef Tea Salad

    2 ounces sliced turkey pastrami

    2 ounces sliced or shredded cooked chicken breast

    2 chopped hard-boiled egg whites

    2 ounces crumbled reduced-fat feta cheese (about ½ cup)

    1 medium Roma tomato, sliced

    ½ cup chopped cucumber

    ½ cup chopped carrots

    ½ cup chopped jicama

    ¼ cup chopped celery

    Sprinkle of any Tea Rub you like (pages 189 to 190)

    8 ounces or as much as you like of your favorite lettuce or spring mix

    Tea Salad Dressing (page 191) or Tea Tomato-Seed Salad Dressing
       (page 191)

Combine everything in a salad bowl and toss gently.

Serves 4

NUTRITION PER SERVING (WITH DRESSING): *calories 220, fat 11g, protein 20g, carb 10g*

DAY 12

Orange Spice Cake Hot Todtea

    Orange Spice Rooibos tisane* to cover the bottom of a teapot or 1 bag
       orange-flavored tea

    1 teaspoon agave nectar or any honey, mixed with 1 tablespoon of hot water

    1 cup filtered water, boiled

    1 tablespoon fat- and sugar-free whipped topping (optional)

Combine the tea and agave nectar in a teapot or cup. Add the water and steep for 3 to 4 minutes and serve hot with whipped topping, if desired.

*If you do not have the Orange Spice Rooibos, use any plain Black Tea or Rooibos tisane and add 1 tablespoon grated orange zest and a pinch of ground cinnamon to the steeping.

If you desire a Frostea, add the brewed tea mixture over ice in a blender and blend to your desired thickness. Serve with whipped topping, if desired. Resteep the loose or bagged tea.

Serves 1
NUTRITION PER SERVING: *calories 35, fat 0 g, protein 1 g, carb 8 g*
WITH 1 TABLESPOON WHIPPED TOPPING: *calories 40, fat 0 g, protein 1 g, carb 10*

Oven-Roasted Tea Tomatoes

1 pound cherry tomatoes

2 tablespoons olive oil

2 tablespoons balsamic vinegar

1 teaspoon ground black pepper

¼ teaspoon finely ground dry tea of your choice

Heat the oven to 375 degrees.

Combine the tomatoes, olive oil, vinegar, pepper, and tea in a baking dish that will hold the tomatoes in one layer. Bake until tomatoes start to split, approximately 25 minutes. Serve hot, warm, at room temperature, or cold.

Servings 4
NUTRITION PER SERVING: *calories 100, fat 7 g, protein 3 g, carb 7 g*

Tea Wild Rice

One 7-ounce box wild rice (any brand)
¼ teaspoon finely ground dry oolong tea

Follow the package directions, substituting tea for salt in recipe.

Serves 4
NUTRITION PER SERVING: *calories 170, fat 0 g, protein 4 g, carb 38 g*

Key Lime Pie Frostea

Any lemon- or lime-flavored tea or tisane* to cover the bottom of a tea pot or
    1 bag lemon- or lime-flavored tea
1 teaspoon agave nectar or any honey, mixed with 1 tablespoon hot water
1 cup filtered water, boiled
Ice to fill a blender

Combine the tea and agave nectar in a teapot or cup. Add the water and steep for 3 minutes. Strain the brewed tea mixture over the ice in a blender and blend to your desired thickness. Serve. Resteep the loose or bagged tea.

*If you do not have Lemon- or Lime-Flavored Tea or Rooibos tisane, use any plain Tea or tisane and add 2 tablespoons fresh lemon or lime juice to the steeping.

Can also be served hot.

Serves 1
NUTRITION PER SERVING: *calories 30, fat 0 g, protein 1 g, carb 8 g*

DAY 13

Strawberry Pie Green Tea Hot Todtea

Strawberry Pie Green Tea* to cover the bottom of a teapot or 1 bag
    strawberry-flavored tea

1 Teaspoon agave nectar or any honey, mixed with 1 tablespoon hot water

1 cup filtered water, boiled

1 tablespoon fat- and sugar-free whipped topping (optional)

Combine the tea and agave nectar in a teapot or cup. Add the water and steep for 2 minutes. Strain and serve hot with whipped topping, if desired.

*If you do not have the Strawberry Pie Green Tea, use any plain Tea or Rooibos tisane and add 1 teaspoon chopped fresh or dried strawberries to the steeping.

If you desire a Frostea, strain the brewed tea mixture over ice in a blender and blend to your desired thickness. Serve with whipped topping, if desired. Resteep the loose or bagged tea.

Serves 1

NUTRITION PER SERVING: *calories 30, fat 0 g, protein 1 g, carb 7 g*

WITH 1 TABLESPOON WHIPPED TOPPING: *calories: 40, fat 0 g, protein 1 g, carb 9 g*

Chinese Tea Chicken Salad

2 whole skinless, boneless chicken breasts (about 1 pound)

*2 teaspoons Chicken Tea Rub (page 189) or add ¼ teaspoon any finely
    ground dry tea to a chicken seasoning you love*

½ cup chopped green bell pepper

1 tablespoon orange juice

1 tablespoon orange pulp

2 pinches any finely ground dry tea

½ head lettuce of your choice, chopped

1 tablespoon sesame seeds

Massage the chicken with Chicken Tea Rub. Cut the chicken into small pieces. Combine the chicken, bell pepper, orange juice and pulp, and dry tea in a large nonstick skillet.

Cook until the chicken turns white and is firm to the touch. Place the chopped lettuce in a large bowl. Drain off any liquid and scoop the chicken and pepper mixture over the lettuce. Garnish with sesame seeds.

Serves 4

NUTRITION PER SERVING: *calories 186, fat 4g, protein 30g, carb 7g*

Tea Turkey Florentine

Two 10-ounce packages frozen spinach, thawed

1 medium lemon

1 pound turkey breast cutlets

Olive oil cooking spray

2 tablespoons all-purpose flour

2 teaspoons Chicken Tea Rub (page 189) or ¼ teaspoon any finely ground dry
  tea added to your best chicken seasoning

2 tablespoons olive oil

½ cup white wine

Squeeze all the liquid out of the spinach. Grate to zest of the lemon, then cut the lemon in half and squeeze the juice.

Spray both sides of each cutlet with olive oil cooking spray. Place the flour, 1 teaspoon of the Tea Rub, and the cutlets in a large resealable plastic bag. Shake the bag to evenly coat the cutlets. Heat 1 tablespoon of the olive oil in a large skillet over medium heat. Brown the cutlets on both sides until cooked through. Remove from the pan and keep warm.

Add the white wine and cook for a few minutes, scraping up any browned bits. Add remaining olive oil. Add the spinach. Stir in the remaining Tea Rub and the lemon juice and zest. Cook for a few minutes, until the spinach is heated through. Stir well to ensure all the flavors have incorporated. Place the turkey cutlets over the spinach and serve.

Serves 4

NUTRITION PER SERVING: *calories 250, fat 8g, protein 33g, carb 13g*

Blueberry Tea Sauce

2 tablespoons brewed blueberry tea or any brewed tea you love

Grated zest of ½ lemon

1 cup blueberries

1 teaspoon cornstarch

1 teaspoon lemon juice

1 teaspoon sugar

½ teaspoon vanilla extract

Combine 1 tablespoon brewed tea, the lemon zest, and the blueberries in a small saucepan. Bring to a boil.

In a small bowl, combine the remaining brewed tea, the cornstarch, lemon juice, sugar, and vanilla. Stir until the cornstarch is dissolved. Add to saucepan and allow to come to a boil one more time. Reduce heat and stir until slightly thickened. Remove from heat and allow to cool.

May be served warm or chilled and with any fruit you love.

Serves 4

NUTRITION PER SERVING: *calories 30, fat 0g, protein 0g, carb 8g*

DAY 14

Tea-Infused Blueberries

¼ cup your favorite hot brewed fruit tea

1 cup fresh blueberries

¼ teaspoon honey (optional)

Pour the hot tea over the blueberries. Stir in the honey, if desired.

Serves 1

NUTRITION PER SERVING (WITHOUT HONEY): *calories 80, fat 1g, protein 1g, carb 23g*

Pineapple Upside-Down Cake Hot Todtea

Green Tea with Pineapple* to cover the bottom of a teapot or 1 bag

  pineapple-flavored tea

1 teaspoon agave nectar or any honey, mixed with 1 tablespoon of hot water

1 cup filtered water, boiled

1 tablespoon sugar-free whipped topping (optional)

Combine the tea and agave nectar in a tea pot or cup. Add the water and steep for 3 to 4 minutes. Strain and serve hot with whipped topping, if desired.

*If you do not have the Green Tea with Pineapple, use any plain green tea or Rooibos tisane and add 1 teaspoon chopped dried or fresh pineapple to the steeping.

If you desire a Frostea, strain the brewed tea mixture over ice in a blender and blend to your desired thickness. Serve with whipped topping, if desired. Resteep the loose or bagged tea.

Serves 1

NUTRITION PER SERVING: *calories 35, fat 0 g, protein 1 g, carb 8 g*

WITH 1 TABLESPOON WHIPPED TOPPING: *calories 40, fat 0 g, protein 1 g, carb 9 g*

Turkey Bacon–Egg Tea Salad Sandwich

1 slice turkey bacon

4 hard-boiled egg whites, chopped

¼ cup brewed white or green tea

1 large tomato or 7 cherry tomatoes, chopped

1 green onion (scallion), trimmed and chopped

2 slices multigrain bread

Cook the turkey bacon to desired crispness and chop. Combine in a medium bowl with the egg whites, brewed tea, tomatoes, and green onion. Serve on the bread as one closed or two open-face sandwiches.

Serves 1

NUTRITION PER SERVING: *calories 370, fat 8 g, protein 31 g, carb 44 g*

Grilled Tea-Marinated Chops

2 tablespoons any brewed fruit-flavored tea

½ teaspoon brown sugar

1 teaspoon ground cinnamon

1 tablespoon Dijon mustard

1 teaspoon ground black pepper

1 teaspoon ground ginger

Four 4-ounce center cut boneless pork or lamb chops, well trimmed

In a small bowl, stir together the brewed tea, brown sugar, cinnamon, mustard, pepper, and ginger. Pour the mixture into a large resealable plastic bag. Add the chops. Allow to sit in the refrigerator overnight.

Heat a grill pan or barbecue to medium-hot. Remove the chops from the bag. Discard the marinade.

Grill the chops until browned on both sides and cooked to your desired doneness. Remove from heat and cover loosely. Allow to rest for 15 minutes before serving.

Serves 4

NUTRITION PER SERVING: *calories 140, fat 6 g, protein 20 g, carb 2 g*

TEABouleh

1 teaspoon your favorite dry tea

1½ cups filtered water, boiled

1 cup bulgar wheat

¼ cup fresh lemon juice

1 tablespoon olive oil

1 unpeeled English cucumber, seeded and chopped into medium pieces

2 cups cherry tomatoes, sliced in half

1 cup chopped fresh parsley

1 cup chopped green onions (scallions)

½ cup chopped fresh mint

   1 teaspoon kosher salt

   1 teaspoon ground pepper

Combine the tea and water and allow to steep for 3 minutes.

In a large bowl, combine the bulgar wheat, lemon juice, and olive oil. Strain the brewed tea over this mixture. Stir. Set aside and allow to sit at room temperature for 1 hour.

Add the cucumber, tomatoes, parsley, green onions, mint, salt, and pepper. Stir well. The TEABouleh may be served at room temperature or refrigerated.

Serves 4

NUTRITION PER SERVING: *calories 130, fat 3g, protein 5g, carb 25g*

Tea Apple Sauce

   2 small apples, peeled, cored, and chopped

   2 tablespoons lemon juice

   2 tablespoons any brewed tea

   2 droppers liquid stevia, or any sugar substitute equivalent to 2 teaspoons sugar

   ½ teaspoon cinnamon

Combine the apples, lemon juice, and brewed tea to a blender. Process until smooth. Stir in the stevia and cinnamon. Refrigerate and serve chilled.

Serves 2

NUTRITION PER ¾-CUP SERVING: *calories 70, fat 0g, protein 0g, carb 18g*

PART 3 ✳ QUICK & EASY RECIPES

Quick & Easy Tea-Infused Yogurt or Cottage Cheese

   2 cups nonfat milk

   ¼ teaspoon ground cinnamon

   3 tablespoons dry Masala Chai or any other dry tea or tisane you love

1 dropper liquid stevia (optional)

2 cups plain nonfat yogurt or one 16-ounce container cottage cheese

Bring the milk, cinnamon, and dry Masala Chai to a boil in a medium saucepan. Lower to a simmer. Continue cooking, stirring the mixture frequently, until the tea and cinnamon mix thoroughly (about 3 minutes). Remove from the heat and stir in the stevia, if using. Allow to settle. Strain the leaves from the mixture. This could be done the night before. Refrigerate.

Place 4 to 6 ounces of yogurt or cottage cheese on your plate, cover with sauce.

Serves 3

NUTRITION PER SERVING: *calories 130, fat 0g, protein 12g, carb 23g*

Quick & Easy Parmesan-Bacon–Egg White Tea Scramble

2 cups filtered water

1 tablespoon any dry green tea

1 piece low-sodium turkey bacon

½ cup sliced crimini or button mushrooms

½ cup chopped bell pepper, any color

1 cup loosely packed baby spinach

3 egg whites

¼ teaspoon ground black pepper

Pinch of red pepper flakes (optional)

2 tablespoons grated nonfat Parmesan cheese

Bring the filtered water to a boil. In another pot place the tea at the bottom and add the now less than boiling water and steep for 3 minutes. Strain. You can resteep the leaves.

Set 2 tablespoons of the brewed tea aside to cool. Enjoy the rest of the tea while preparing your scramble.

Chop the turkey bacon and place in a nonstick skillet. Cook over medium heat until about half done. Add the mushrooms. If there is not enough fat from the bacon, you can add a little brewed tea to the pan. Add the bell peppers and cook for a few minutes. Add the spinach and cook until wilted.

In a small bowl, lightly whisk the egg whites, 2 tablespoons of brewed tea, pepper, and red pepper flakes, if using. Add the egg mixture to the pan and cook, stirring, until done to your taste. Stir in the cheese just before serving.

Serves 1

NUTRITION PER SERVING: *calories 290, fat 8 g, protein 32 g, carb 23 g*

Quick & Easy Tea Omelet with Spinach and Turkey Bacon

> *3 egg whites*
> *½ cup brewed tea (any oolong, Assam, or other black tea)*
> *Dash of Tabasco sauce*
> *Ground pepper*
> *2 cups loosely packed baby spinach*
> *1 medium roma tomato, seeded and chopped*
> *3 slices turkey bacon*

Whisk together the egg whites, 2 tablespoons of the brewed tea, the Tabasco, and a pinch of pepper. In medium nonstick skillet, wilt the spinach in the remaining brewed tea. Add the tomato and cook for a few minutes allowing the flavors to marry. Remove the spinach-tomato mixture from pan.

Over medium heat, cook the bacon in the sauce pan. Remove and cut into bite-size pieces.

Add the egg whites to the pan and cook undisturbed until set. Place the spinach-tomato mixture and turkey bacon on half of the omelet. Fold the other side over. Keep over the heat just until heated through.

Serves 1

NUTRITION PER SERVING: *calories 220, fat 6 g, protein 31 g, carb 11 g*

Quick & Easy Egg White–Tea Omelet

> 3 egg whites
> ½ teaspoon finely ground dry tea
> 1 teaspoon minced fresh parsley
> Salt and pepper
> ½ cup chopped veggies*
> 1 tablespoon reduced-fat feta, nonfat ricotta, cottage cheese, or chopped
>   string cheese

Beat the egg whites with the dry tea, parsley, and salt and pepper to taste. Stir in the vegetables and cheese. Heat a medium nonstick skillet over medium heat. Pour in the mixture and cook on one side until golden. Flip and cook the other side.

*Use any cooked veggies that are in your fridge, spinach, mushrooms, peppers, zucchini, onions, or any raw veggies you love.

Serves: 1
NUTRITION PER SERVING: *calories 50, fat 0g, protein 0g, carb 12g*

Quick & Easy Broccoli Tea Soup

> 1 tablespoon olive oil
> 1 medium onion, sliced
> 1 pound broccoli florets
> 2 cups brewed oolong tea
> 3 cups low-sodium chicken or vegetable broth
> Ground black pepper
> ¼ cup grated Parmesan cheese

Heat the olive oil in a large saucepan. Add the onion and cook until translucent, approximately 5 minutes. Add the broccoli, brewed tea, and broth. Cook over medium to low heat until broccoli is tender, approximately 20 minutes. Blend in small batches in a blender. Hold a towel over the lid of the blender to prevent splatter. Reheat. Season the soup to taste with the black pepper. Serve with a sprinkling of Parmesan cheese.

Serves 6
NUTRITION PER SERVING: *calories 80, fat 4 g, protein 6 g, carb 7 g*

Quick & Easy Tea Gazpacho

1 medium red bell pepper, seeded and chopped

1 medium green bell pepper, seeded and chopped

1 large cucumber, peeled, seeded, and chopped

One 28-ounce can chopped tomatoes, with their juice

1 medium onion, chopped

2 cloves garlic, chopped

3 tablespoons red wine vinegar

1 tablespoon olive oil

1 teaspoon finely ground dry oolong tea

4 drops Tabasco sauce

Salt and ground pepper

Set aside one quarter of the bell peppers and cucumber to use as garnish.

Place the tomatoes, onions, the remaining bell peppers, cucumber, garlic, vinegar, oil, and Tabasco in a food processor and process until the desired consistency. It is always good to have a little texture.

Transfer the soup to a container, cover, and refrigerate for a few hours or overnight. If the soup is too thick, thin it out with cold-brewed Oolong Tea. Adjust the seasoning to taste.

Serve chilled, garnished with the reserved chopped peppers and cucumber.

Serves 4
NUTRITION PER SERVING: *calories 180, fat .5 g, protein 9 g, carb 38 g*

Quick & Easy Tea Crab Salad in Endive Leaves

1 head Belgian endive

¼ pound fresh crabmeat

¼ cup brewed Key Lime Pie Tea or any tea you love

1 tablespoon capers, rinsed and drained

1 tablespoon chopped fresh basil

1 tablespoon chopped green onions (scallions)

½ teaspoon ground black pepper

Separate the endive leaves and place on a serving platter. Pick through the crabmeat to ensure that all the shell has been removed. In a bowl, combine the crabmeat with the brewed tea, capers, basil, green onions, and pepper. Spoon into the endive leaves.

Serves 1

NUTRITION PER SERVING: *calories 110, fat 1 g, protein 21 g, carb 4 g*

Quick & Easy Tea Hummus with Whole-Wheat Pita

Two 15-ounce cans garbanzo beans (chickpeas), drained

¼ cup tahini paste

2 cloves garlic, chopped

½ teaspoon kosher salt

½ teaspoon ground black pepper

¼ teaspoon red pepper flakes

½ cup brewed Key Lime Pie Tea (or other lemon-flavored tea)

8 whole-wheat pitas

Heat the oven to 350 degrees F.

Place the garbanzo beans, tahini, garlic, salt, pepper, and red pepper flakes in the bowl of a food processor. Add half of the brewed tea. Blend, adding remaining brewed tea slowly until the hummus is the desired consistency. Season to taste with more salt and/or pepper if needed.

Cut the pita into quarters. Warm the pita for a few minutes in the oven.

Serves 16

NUTRITION PER SERVING: *calories 130, fat 3.5 g, protein 6 g, carb 21 g*

Quick & Easy Pear and Goat Cheese Tea Salad

1 firm Bartlett or Bosc pear

¼ cup balsamic vinegar

2 heads romaine lettuce

4 ounces soft goat cheese (about 1 cup)

1 tablespoon chopped walnuts

¼ teaspoon kosher salt

½ teaspoon ground black pepper

¼ teaspoon finely ground dry green tea

2 tablespoons olive oil

Slice the pear into thin slices. Pour a little of the vinegar over the pear to prevent it from discoloring; the flavor of the vinegar will infuse into the pear. Break the lettuce into bite-size pieces and place in a large salad bowl. Cut or crumble the cheese into small pieces and add to the lettuce. Add the sliced pear and walnuts.

Mix together the salt, pepper, dry tea, olive oil and remainder of the balsamic vinegar. Toss together with the salad.

Serves 4

NUTRITION PER SERVING: *calories 230, fat 14 g, protein 9 g, carb 20 g*

Quick & Easy Spicy Veggie Tea Pasta

2 tablespoons olive oil

1 pound crimini mushrooms, sliced

One 14-ounce can chopped tomatoes

2 cups broccoli florets

2 cups loosely packed spinach leaves

1 teaspoon ground black pepper

1 teaspoon kosher salt

½ teaspoon ground red pepper

Pinch of red pepper flakes

1 teaspoon dry oolong tea

½ of a 12- to 14.5-ounce package multigrain penne pasta

½ cup grated Parmesan cheese

Bring a large saucepan of water to a boil.

Meanwhile, heat the olive oil in a large nonstick skillet over medium heat. Sauté the mushrooms in the olive oil until soft. A little water can be added once the olive oil is absorbed. Add the tomatoes and simmer.

Boil or microwave the broccoli for just a few minutes to soften slightly. Add to the skillet. Add the spinach and stir to wilt. Stir in the black pepper, salt, ground red pepper, and pepper flakes.

Add the dry tea to the boiling water. Cook the penne for 6 minutes, just until cooked through. Drain the penne.

Add the pasta to the pan. Stir. Add the Parmesan cheese and serve.

Grilled chicken or steak can be added to this recipe.

Serves 4

NUTRITION PER SERVING: *calories 360, fat 11 g, protein 14 g, carb 53 g*

Quick & Easy Tea-Boiled Shrimp

> Filtered water
>
> ½ teaspoon kosher salt
>
> ¼ teaspoon black pepper
>
> 1 tablespoon dry oolong tea or other tea you love
>
> 1 pound fresh or frozen peeled, deveined shrimp (thawed if frozen)
>
> 2 tablespoons extra virgin olive oil
>
> 1 small to medium clove garlic, minced
>
> 3 tablespoons fresh lemon juice

Fill large saucepan or deep skillet with filtered water. Bring to a boil and add the salt, pepper, and dry tea. Add the shrimp and remove from the heat. Let the shrimp sit until you see them turning pink. While the shrimp are cooking, in a medium saucepan, heat the olive oil and garlic. Do not let the garlic burn. Remove from the heat and add the lemon juice. Drain the shrimp.*

Put the shrimp in a serving bowl, toss with the sauce, and serve.

*I eat the tea leaves with the shrimp as they add a great flavor, or you can remove them by rinsing them under water.

Serves 4

NUTRITION PER SERVING: *calories 190, fat 9 g, protein 24 g, carb 3 g*

Quick & Easy Tea Corn on the Cob

> 2 quarts filtered water
>
> 2 tablespoons dry green tea
>
> ¼ teaspoon salt
>
> ¼ teaspoon ground pepper
>
> 4 large ears fresh corn, shucked, silk removed (organic if possible)

Bring the filtered water to a boil in a large saucepan. Add the dry tea, salt, and pepper to the water. Add corn and cook to desired firmness. Remove and serve.

Serves: 4

NUTRITION PER SERVING: *calories 130, fat 1 g, protein 6 g, carb 29 g*

Quick & Easy Tea Oven-Poached Salmon

1 clove garlic

1 tablespoon of your favorite dried fruit tea

3 cups filtered water

½ teaspoon grated or minced fresh ginger

Four 4-ounce salmon fillets

1 lemon, sliced

Preheat the oven to 350 degrees F.

Combine the garlic, dry tea, filtered water, and ginger in a medium saucepan and bring to a boil. Reduce the heat and simmer for 5 minutes. Pour the poaching liquid into a baking dish fitted with a rack; the liquid should not reach the rack.

Place the salmon fillets on the rack and cover with the lemon slices. Place the baking pan carefully in the oven and bake until cooked through, approximately 20 minutes. The fish is done when it flakes easily with a fork.

Serves: 4

NUTRITION PER SERVING: *calories 190, fat 6 g, protein 32 g, carb 1 g*

PART 4 ✴ ADDITIONAL RECIPES

SOUP

Onion Tea Soup

2 tablespoons olive oil

4 large onions, sliced thin

2 cups low-sodium chicken broth

4 cups brewed tea (golden Assam, or any oolong tea)

1 bay leaf

1 teaspoon ground black pepper

2 teaspoons Worcestershire sauce

1 tablespoon Sherry or brandy

1 tablespoon grated Parmesan cheese

4 thin slices French bread (1 ounce each)

Heat the olive oil in a large saucepan. Add the onions and sauté until translucent, 3 to 4 minutes. Add the chicken broth, brewed tea, bay leaf, pepper, and Worcestershire sauce. Bring to a boil. Lower the heat and simmer for 30 minutes. Remove the bay leaf. Add the Sherry or brandy.

While the soup is simmering, heat the oven to 400 degrees F. Sprinkle the Parmesan cheese over the bread and place on a baking sheet. Bake for 15 minutes, or until crisp and the cheese has melted.

Place a slice of toast in the bottom of each of four soup bowls and pour one quarter of the soup over each.

Serves 4
NUTRITION PER SERVING (SOUP ONLY): *calories 140, fat 7g, protein 4g, carb 16g*

SIDE DISHES

French Bread with Parmesan (carb option)

1 tablespoon grated Parmesan cheese

4 thin slices French bread

Heat the oven to 400 degrees F. Place the bread on a baking sheet. Sprinkle the Parmesan cheese over the bread. Bake for 15 minutes, or until crisp and the cheese has melted.

Serves 4
NUTRITION PER SERVING: *calories 90, fat 1.5g, protein 3g, carb 16g*

Ayurvedic Tomato-Cucumber Tea Yogurt

1 teaspoon cumin seeds

1 teaspoon your favorite dry chai or any other dry tea

1 cup Greek nonfat yogurt or your favorite nonfat yogurt

1½ large tomatoes, peeled, seeded,* and cut into small pieces

½ cup peeled, seeded, diced Japanese or English cucumber

Kosher salt and pepper

In a small dry skillet, roast the cumin seeds, stirring, until lightly brown and you begin to smell the aroma. Add the dry tea and roast for 1 minute more over low heat. Remove from the heat and place in a blender or a mortar and grind the cumin and tea until powdered.

Drain the yogurt of any moisture.

In a medium bowl, combine the tomato and cucumber with salt and pepper to taste. Stir in the tea-cumin powder. Add the yogurt and mix evenly. Cover and refrigerate until needed. Drain any liquid that may have accumulated before serving.

*Use the seeds for Tea Tomato-Seed Salad Dressing.

Serves 4

NUTRITION PER SERVING: *calories 50, fat 0 g, protein 6 g, carb 6 g*

French Tea Ratatouille

1 tablespoon extra virgin olive oil

2 small eggplants (preferably Japanese), halved lengthwise

1 small to medium clove garlic, minced

3 cups filtered water

1 tablespoon dry oolong tea

2 tomatoes, peeled and chopped coarsely

1 onion, chopped

1 cup chopped zucchini

¼ *teaspoon kosher salt*

¼ *teaspoon ground black pepper*

1 *tablespoon fresh lemon juice*

Heat the oven to 350 degrees F.

Heat the olive oil in a medium skillet. Add the eggplant skin side down and cook until the skin softens. Sprinkle the garlic around the eggplant and cook until the garlic browns lightly. Remove from the heat.

Bring the filtered water to a boil and set aside for a minute. Add the dry oolong tea and brew for 3 minutes.

Place the eggplant skin side down in a large baking dish. Cover with the tomatoes, onions, and zucchini. Sprinkle with the salt and pepper, and pour in the tea (including the leaves). Bake for 30 minutes, or until the desired tenderness of the vegetables is reached. Remove from the oven and let stand for 15 minutes. Pour the lemon juice on top and serve.

Serves: 4

NUTRITION PER SERVING: *calories 140, fat 4.5 g, protein 5 g, carb 23 g*

ENTREES

Cajun Tea Salmon Fillets

1 *teaspoon finely ground dry Lapsang Souchong Black Tea or any black tea you love*

1 *tablespoon paprika*

1 *teaspoon dried sage*

½ *teaspoon onion powder*

½ *teaspoon cayenne pepper*

½ *teaspoon kosher salt*

½ *teaspoon ground pepper*

½ *teaspoon garlic powder*

1 teaspoon extra virgin olive oil

Four 4-ounce salmon fillets

In a small bowl, combine the dry tea, paprika, sage, onion powder, cayenne pepper, salt, pepper, and garlic powder. Sprinkle the flesh side of the salmon heavily with the spices. Heat the olive oil in a large skillet over medium-high heat. When the oil is hot, add the fillets skin side down. Turn heat down to medium. Cook on until nicely browned, 3 to 4 minutes. Carefully turn over and cook 3 to 4 minutes longer.

Serves 4

NUTRITION PER SERVING: *calories 150, fat 5 g, protein 23 g, carb 1 g*

Chicken Tea Soft Tacos

Cooking Spray

1 pound chicken tenders

1 teaspoon Chicken Tea Rub (page 189), finely ground or ¼ teaspoon tea you love added to chicken seasoning

4 dashes of Tabasco sauce

Juice of 1 lime

3 small zucchini, sliced lengthwise into planks

1 red bell pepper, seeded and sliced

1 red onion, sliced crosswise

2 tablespoons olive oil

8 small whole-wheat tortillas

1 tablespoon chopped cilantro

Spray a grill pan with a cooking spray. Heat over medium-high heat.

Season the chicken with the Chicken Tea Rub, Tabasco, and half of the lime juice. Cook the chicken until well browned on all sides. Remove from pan and set aside.

Drizzle the zucchini, red bell pepper, and onion with the olive oil. Cook in the grill pan until lightly browned on both sides. Remove from the pan and sprinkle with the remaining lime juice. Slice the chicken tenders into strips. Warm the tortillas. Divide the chicken and vegetables among the tortillas. Sprinkle with the chopped cilantro.

Serves 4

NUTRITION PER SERVING: *calories 370, fat 10 g, protein 33 g, carb 48 g,*

Tea Chicken Piccata

> 2 tablespoons all-purpose flour
>
> 1 teaspoon ground pepper
>
> ½ teaspoon kosher salt
>
> ¼ teaspoon finely ground dry oolong tea
>
> 1 pound skinless, boneless chicken breast halves
>
> 2 tablespoons olive oil
>
> Juice of 2 lemons
>
> ½ cup white wine

Mix the flour, pepper, salt, and dry tea in a large resealable plastic bag. Add the chicken, seal the bag, and shake until the chicken is evenly coated.

Heat the olive oil over medium heat in a large nonstick skillet. Place the chicken into the pan and cook until browned on both sides, approximately 3 minutes per side. Remove the chicken from the pan and place on a sheet of paper towel to absorb any excess oil. Add the lemon juice and white wine to the pan. Cook, scraping up any brown bits, until the sauce reduces by half. Add the chicken back into the pan. Simmer for 5 minutes before serving.

This is delicious served over cauliflower tea mash.

Serves 4

NUTRITION PER SERVING: *calories 230, fat 8 g, protein 27 g, carb 8 g*

Eggplant and Sun-Dried Tomato Tea Chicken

> 2 tablespoons olive oil
>
> 1 medium red onion, sliced
>
> 2 cloves garlic, chopped

1 pound skinless, boneless chicken breast halves

1 teaspoon Chicken or Vegetable Tea Rub or ¼ teaspoon finely ground dry
tea you love added to any chicken seasoning

½ teaspoon dried oregano

Juice of ½ lemon

3 Japanese eggplants, sliced into ½-inch rounds

½ cup brewed tea you love, or more as needed

1 tablespoon chopped sun-dried tomatoes (oil packed)

Grated zest of ½ lemon

1 teaspoon chopped fresh basil

Heat the olive oil in a large nonstick skillet over medium-high heat. Add the onion and garlic and cook until softened. Remove from the pan and set aside.

Season the chicken with the Chicken Tea Rub, oregano, and lemon juice. Place in the pan and cook until brown on both sides. Add the chicken to the onion.

Place the eggplant in the pan. Add ½ cup brewed tea and cook until soft. Sprinkle with a pinch of Chicken or Vegetable Tea Rub. Add the sun-dried tomatoes and cook for just a few minutes to allow flavors to blend. You can add a few tablespoons of brewed tea to the pan if you feel that you need more liquid.

Add the chicken and onion back to the pan and cook until heated through. Add the lemon zest and chopped basil. Place on a platter and serve.

Serves 4
NUTRITION PER SERVING: *calories 310, fat 9 g, protein 31 g, carb 28 g*

Artichoke Tea Chicken

2 teaspoons any dry green tea

2 tablespoons all-purpose flour

½ teaspoon kosher salt

1 teaspoon ground black pepper

1½ pounds skinless, boneless chicken breast halves

2 tablespoons olive oil

½ cup white wine

One 14-ounce can artichoke hearts, drained and quartered

8 pieces sun-dried tomatoes (drained if oil-packed)

8 chopped pitted Kalamata olives

1 tablespoon chopped basil or 1 teaspoon dry

1 tablespoon chopped fresh thyme or 1 teaspoon dry

¼ teaspoon red pepper flakes

1 tablespoon capers, rinsed and drained

Boil 1 cup water. Add the dry tea and steep for 10 minutes.

Place the flour, salt, and black pepper in a large resealable plastic bag. Add the chicken and shake until evenly coated. In a large skillet, heat the olive oil over medium-high heat. Brown the chicken lightly on each side. Remove from the pan. Add the white wine to the pan to deglaze it, scraping up any browned bits. Strain the tea into the skillet and cook for 10 minutes.

Add the artichokes, tomatoes, olives, basil, thyme, and red pepper flakes. Simmer for 10 minutes. Add the chicken back into the pan. Stir until well covered. Cook for approximately 20 minutes, adding the capers about 5 minutes before serving.

This chicken may be baked in a 350 degree F oven for 30 minutes instead of on the stove top, if preferred.

Serves 6

NUTRITION PER SERVING: *calories 360, fat 8 g, protein 28 g, carb 46 g*

Apricot-Ginger Black Tea Chicken Breasts

1 cup dried or fresh apricots, cut into small pieces (pitted if fresh)

2 tablespoons finely chopped fresh ginger

2 tablespoons dry Earl Grey Tea or your favorite dry tea

2 tablespoons soy sauce

2 cloves garlic

1 teaspoon extra virgin olive oil

Four 4-ounce skinless, boneless chicken breast halves

2 tablespoons chopped cilantro

Heat the oven to 375 degrees F.

Combine the apricots, ginger, dry tea, soy sauce, and garlic in the bowl of a food processor and process until a smooth puree.

Brush the chicken breasts with the olive oil. Place them skin side down in an ovenproof nonstick skillet and cook over medium-high heat until the skin is lightly browned. Turn over and brown the other side. Brush the tea mixture generously onto that side, then turn over and brush it generously on the skin. Place the skillet in the oven and bake for 30 to 40 minutes, or until the apricot glaze is browned but not burnt.

Remove from the oven, plate, sprinkle the top with the cilantro, and serve.

Serves 4

NUTRITION PER SERVING: *calories 260, fat 3g, protein 30g, carb 27g*

Special Plum Tea Pork or Beef Loin

3 cloves garlic, chopped

1 tablespoon chopped fresh rosemary

1 tablespoon chopped fresh thyme

1 teaspoon ground black pepper

1 teaspoon finely grated lemon zest

*1 tablespoon finely ground dry Plum Oolong Tea or 2 to 3 tablespoons any
dry tea you love mixed with 1 teaspoon chopped dried plums and ground
together*

1 tablespoon extra virgin olive oil

1 tablespoon Dijon mustard

2½ pounds boneless pork loin

Take the meat out of the refrigerator 30 minutes before you will cook it. Preheat the oven to 350 degrees F.

In a small bowl, mix the garlic, rosemary, thyme, pepper, lemon zest, and dry tea with the olive oil and mustard until it forms a paste. Rub the mixture all over the meat. Place in a roasting pan and roast for 1 to 1½ hours, or until internal temperature reaches 150 degrees F. Cover loosely and allow to rest for 20 minutes before slicing and serving.

If you do not eat pork, substitute trimmed beef tenderloin.

Serves 8
NUTRITION PER SERVING: *calories 230, fat 12 g, protein 27 g, carb 2 g*

DESSERTS

Apple Tea Cobbler

Cooking spray
5 cups sliced Fuji or any of your favorite apples
5 cups sliced Granny Smith apples
2 tablespoons orange juice
¼ cup your favorite brewed fruit tea
½ cup whole-wheat flour
1 teaspoon grated orange zest
2 tablespoon ground cinnamon
6 tablespoons granulated sugar substitute
½ cup old-fashioned oats
½ cup fat-free margarine spread

Preheat oven to 350 degrees F. Lightly coat a 13- by 9-inch baking dish with cooking spray.

Combine the apples in a large bowl. Pour the orange juice and brewed tea over the apples and toss to coat. In a small bowl, combine ¼ cup of flour, the orange zest, 1 tablespoon of the cinnamon, and 2 tablespoons of the sugar substitute. Toss gently with the apples. Spread in the prepared baking dish.

Combine the remaining flour, sugar substitute, and cinnamon with the oats and margarine. Stir until crumbly. Sprinkle the topping over the apples.

Bake for approximately 50 minutes, until the apples are fork-tender and bubbling, and the topping is browned.

This cobbler can be made with any fruit or a combination of different fruit.

Serves 12
NUTRITION PER SERVING: *calories 160, fat 8 g, protein 2 g, carb 22 g*

Tea Ice Cubes

Make your ice cubes with your favorite tea instead of water. You will have full-flavored iced tea instead of watered-down tea.

Take a little extra time to make the ice cubes a little more special. Small slices of orange, lemon, or lime added to your ice cube sections before pouring the tea in will look beautiful when frozen and will add extra flavor to your tea as the ice cube melts.

Blueberry Tea Cubes Add 2 blueberries to each section of your ice tray before pouring the tea in. Serves 6 (1 tray of 12 ice cubes) Calories 5, fat 0 g, protein 0 g, carb 1 g.

Orange Tea Cubes Zest an orange into long strips. Add a strip of orange zest to each section of your ice tray. Pour the tea in and freeze. Serves 6. Calories 0, fat 0 g, protein 0 g, carb 1 g.

Strawberry Tea Cubes Add small pieces of strawberry to the sections of the ice tray before freezing. Serves 6. Calories 0, fat 0 g, protein 0 g, carb 0 g.

Apple Tea Cubes Add small chunks of apple with the peel left to your ice cube sections before pouring apple or any fruit tea into the tray. Serves 6. Calories 5, fat 0 g, protein 0 g, carb 1 g.

Ginger Tea Cubes Use a zester that makes long thin strips of ginger to liven up ginger tea ice cubes. Serves 6. Calories 0, fat 0 g, protein 0 g, carb 0 g.

Pineapple Tea Cubes Add small pieces of pineapple to your ice cube trays before filling with the tea. Serves 6. Calories 5, fat 0 g, protein 0 g, carb 1 g.

Have fun with your ice cubes. The options are limitless.

PART 5 ✳ DINNER PARTY FOR FOUR WITH TEA PAIRINGS

STARTER

Grilled Tea Shrimp with Yogurt Curry Sauce
Tea Pairing: Green Oolong Tea

> 2 tablespoons extra virgin olive oil (EVOO)
> 2 teaspoon brewed oolong tea
> ¼ teaspoon kosher salt
> ¼ teaspoon ground black pepper
> ¼ teaspoon red pepper flakes
> 12 large raw shrimp (peeled but keep the tails on)
> Salad greens, for serving

Combine the olive oil, brewed tea, salt, pepper and red pepper flakes in a large resealable plastic bag or bowl. Add the shrimp and allow to marinate for at least 30 minutes in the refrigerator.

Heat a grill pan over high heat. Grill the shrimp until cooked. Serve on salad greens with Yogurt Curry Sauce.

Yogurt Curry Sauce

> 1 cup fat-free Greek yogurt or any plain fat-free yogurt
> ½ teaspoon curry powder

2 teaspoons finely ground dry Key Lime Pie Tea or any dry tea

1 teaspoon chopped chives

Mix all ingredients together and serve with the shrimp.

Serves 4

NUTRITION PER SERVING (WITH SALAD GREENS): *calories 170, fat 10g, protein 14g, carb 6g*

MAIN COURSE

Tea Chicken Marsala-Masala
Tea Pairing: Black Masala Chai

2 tablespoons all-purpose flour

1 teaspoon ground black pepper

8 chicken breast tenders

4 tablespoons olive oil

2 shallots, chopped

12 ounces sliced crimini mushrooms

½ cup Marsala wine

1 cup brewed Masala Chai or any black tea, plus more if needed

1 tablespoon low-fat sour cream

Kosher salt

Place the flour and black pepper in a large plastic bag. Add the chicken and shake to coat evenly.

Heat 2 tablespoons of the olive oil in a large nonstick skillet over medium heat. Add the chicken and cook for approximately 7 minutes each side, until brown. Remove chicken from the pan and set aside. Add the remaining olive oil to the pan. Add the shallots and cook until translucent, about 2 minutes. Add the mushrooms and cook for another 2 minutes. If all liquid is cooked out, do not worry, simply add a little brewed tea.

Add the Marsala wine and cook for 2 minutes. Add the brewed tea. Cook for approximately 8 minutes, until liquid is reduced by one third. Add the sour cream and stir until smooth. Taste sauce and adjust seasonings, adding a little salt if needed.

Return the chicken to the pan and reheat a few minutes over low heat. Serve over Currant Tea Couscous.

Serves 4
NUTRITION PER SERVING (CHICKEN AND SAUCE): *calories 240, fat 13g, protein 9g, carb 17g*

Currant Tea Couscous

> 1 to 2 cups brewed Strawberry or Raspberry fruit tea or tisane, or any black
>   tea (according to package directions)
> 1 tablespoon butter
> 1 cup dry instant couscous
> ½ cup currants

In a medium saucepan, bring the brewed tea and butter to a boil. Remove from the heat. Stir in the couscous and currants. Cover and allow to stand for 5 minutes. Fluff with a fork.

Serves 4
NUTRITION PER SERVING: *calories 240, fat 3g, protein 6g, carb 47g*

Oven-Roasted Tea Tomatoes

Prepare the recipe on page 228, using cherry or tear drop tomatoes in a mix of colors, if available. If you like, sprinkle the tomatoes with 1 tablespoon grated Parmesan cheese as soon as you remove them from the oven.

NUTRITION PER SERVING (WITHOUT CHEESE): *calories 100, fat 7g, protein 3g, carb 7g*

DESSERT

Baked Tea Apples

Tea Pairing: Caramel Rooibos Tisane

Prepare the recipe on page 222. These are delicious eaten warm, and elegant served with a sugar-free vanilla pudding or fat-free whipped topping.

NUTRITION PER SERVING (APPLE ONLY): *calories 120, fat 2.5 g, protein 1 g, carb 28 g*

NUTRITION PER SERVING (WITH ½ CUP PUDDING): *calories 229, fat 4 g, protein 13 g, carb 40 g*

NUTRITION PER SERVING (WITH 2 TABLESPOONS FAT-FREE WHIPPED TOPPING): *calories 207, fat 4 g, protein 13 g, carb 35 g*

TEAmmate Profile

Name: **Pam F.**

Age: **39**

Total Weight Loss: **5**

Total Inches Lost: **6.5**

Favorite Tea: **Orange Spice Cake**

I have had a weight problem all of my life. I've tried all kinds of diets—from the Scarsdale diet to the Atkins diet to the liquid diet to Weight Watchers . . . you name it, I've tried it. I usually lose weight in the beginning, but then I get bored with it, and as soon as I go off, the weight comes back, plus.

I have to admit that I went into this program really hoping to lose a lot of weight quickly. Where I got that idea from, I don't know; probably because that is what I was used to reading from other diet books. Anyway, I did not lose a ton of weight in the first few weeks. But I did lose weight and inches, and since I have been doing this program, my skin looks so much better (I have actually been told that I look a lot younger). I have more confidence and I feel so much better—not sluggish like I was before.

The best things that I have learned while doing this program are: 1) I will drink tea for the rest of my life—and will try to get as many other people to drink it as possible; 2) I am more conscious of the things I am eating (and drinking); 3) Exercise is a must in a healthy life (I had hurt my shoulder and did not exercise for the first six weeks, but have been gradually adding it back in. I feel so much better and I have much more energy); 4) Inches are just as important, or more important, than pounds when losing weight.

Anyway, I am so thankful for meeting Dr. Tea and for being included in such a fantastic program with so many great people. I will be talking about this program—and especially about drinking tea—for the rest of my life. I am a changed person (for the better).

12

The History of Tea

The history of tea is long and convoluted. It travels from one country to another, starting in China and working its way around the world in fits and starts, causing revolutions in taste, lifestyle, and, of course, politics. In fact, if tea had not been discovered, the course of world events would have been very different.

No one knows for sure how tea came to be discovered. Legends abound, although there are two that are most famous.

The most popular, and the one that most historians agree might actually have happened, involves the Chinese emperor Shen Nung. He was a skilled leader, a patron of the arts, and a scientist. One of his edicts was that all drinking water be boiled as a hygienic precaution. One day in 2737 BC, as he (or more probably his servant) was boiling his water to drink, some leaves from what we now know as the *Camellia sinensis* plant accidentally blew into the pot. Being the curious scientist he was, Shen Nung decided to taste the liquid and found it very refreshing. And so, tea was born.

The second legend, which comes from Japan, is a bit more gory and a lot more fanciful. This one says that an Indian prince name Bodhidharma was visiting China from India in order to spread Buddhism. He is said to have sat facing the wall at Shaolin Temple meditating without moving for nine years. At some point, he fell asleep while doing so. Supposedly, he became so frustrated by this that he ripped off his eyelids and threw them to the ground. Then, it is said, the deity Quan Yin made the first tea bush sprout on the place where his eyelids fell in order to aid him and all followers of Zen on their path to enlightenment.

Needless to say, I prefer to believe in legend number one.

What follows is a brief, noncomprehensive history of tea facts and fancies, according to history and hearsay.

Tea in Asia

* In its first years, tea was associated with royalty. It is documented that as far back as the twelfth century BC, King Wen of Zhou received tea as a tribute to his reign.

* Until the third century BC, fresh tea leaves were merely boiled in water. Then the drying and processing of the tea leaves into green tea began, and tea consumption began to spread across all of China.

* White tea was produced and was reserved for royalty.

* The earliest credible documented record of tea, chronicled in an ancient Chinese dictionary in 350 AD by noted scholar Kuo Po, described the tea tree and manner of making the beverage. At that time, tea was a bitter-tasting medicinal drink made from raw green tea leaves that were pressed into cakes, roasted, pounded into tiny pieces, boiled in a kettle of water, and flavored with onion, ginger, and orange.

* By the fifth century AD, tea was being used as a medium of exchange. Turkish traders began to bargain for tea on the Mongolian border.

* During the T'ang Dynasty, which lasted from 618–907 AD, powdered tea became the rage. It was often mixed with other ingredients and

brewed, becoming a popular drink throughout China. Caravans carried tea on the Silk Road, trading with India, Turkey, and Russia.

* Between 648 and 749 AD, a Japanese monk named Gyoki brought tea to Japan. He built forty-nine Buddhist temples throughout the country and planted tea bushes at each one. This rare and expensive Japanese tea was enjoyed mostly by priests and royalty.

* In 780 AD, Chinese poet and scholar Lu Yu wrote the *Ch'a Ching,* or "The Classic of Tea," the first comprehensive book about tea, written in exhaustive detail, in which he explained every aspect of tea, from cultivation to preparation techniques to the art of tea appreciation. He began work in 760 and completed the work twenty years later. The book made Lu Yu a celebrity in his time.

* With the advent of Lu Yu's book, tea became extremely popular in China, and in 800 AD tea began to be commercially cultivated.

* In 803 AD, Japanese Buddhist monk Saicho went to China to study Zen Buddhism. He returned home in 805 with fellow monk Eichu, and brought with him tea seeds and the knowledge of creating green tea, presenting it in powdered form and whisking it with bamboo.

* The present-day Japanese tea ceremony (*Cha-no-yu,* or "the hot water for tea") originated in China, and while it died out in China, it continues today in Japan. The Japanese tea ceremony spurred a special type of architecture for "tea houses"; it also promoted geishas to specialize in the presentation of the tea ceremony. Wealthy families took part in tea tournaments, where challengers, hoping to win valuable prizes, competed in identifying various tea blends.

* 1280: Mongolia took over China. The Mongolians were as fond of tea as were the Chinese, and tea drinking becomes more popular among the masses and less popular among the Chinese aristocracy.

* After the fall of the Mongols, the Ming Dynasty (1368–1502) began. Processed loose tea—white, green, oolong, and black—as we know it today was added to hot water. People again began to enjoy tea. The new method of preparation was steeping whole leaves in water. The resulting pale liquid necessitated a lighter color ceramic than was popular in the past. The white and off white tea-ware produced became the style of the time. The first Yixing (ee-HSING) pots were made at this time (Yixing is a region in China known for its purple clay, and the unglazed teapots produced from it).

Tea in Europe

* Dutch navigator Jan Hugo van Linschooten mentions tea for the first time in a 1597 English translation of his travel diaries, in which he refers to tea as "chaa."

* In 1602, the Dutch East India Trading Company was formed, which was the beginning of "world trade" and led to the world's introduction to tea.

* 1610: Green tea was introduced to Holland via trade ships from Java where they picked up tea that had been dropped off by Chinese vessels. Black tea did not replace the green tea until the mid 1700s.

* Tea first came to Russia in 1618 when the Chinese embassy presented some tea to the Czar (which he refused as useless). In the late 1600s, with the Treaty of Nerchinsk, caravan trading began between China and Russia, and camel and horse trains of tea would be taken to the border and exchanged for Russian furs. This journey took about a year and it was here that tea would be infused at night with smoke from the camp fires—and Lapsong Souchong tea was born.

* By 1675, tea was generally used throughout Holland as an everyday drink. Tea made a big splash in France and Germany during this same time, but fell out of favor in place of wine and beer.

* Tea first arrived in Paris in 1636 (twenty-two years before it arrived in England). In the 1670s, Madame de Sévigné, who was a famous gossip and letter writer, wrote to her daughter, "Saw the Princess de Tarente . . . who takes 12 cups of tea every day . . . which, she says, cures all her ills. She assures me that Monsieur de Landgrave drank 40 cups every morning . . . he was dying and it brought him back to life before our eyes. . . ."

* In another letter Madame de Sévigné wrote about a friend of hers who was tired of breaking her precious tea ware due to the heat of the water and one day added cold milk prior to the tea. The dishes did not break and the addition of milk to tea was born. That's right, the English did not invent this.

* Back in Russia in the 1730s, a new tea-drinking tradition began. The Russians used tea concentrate, added hot water, popped in a slice of lemon, and drank the tea through a lump of sugar held between the teeth.

TEASER

Impressions of Tea

Even the art world was influenced by tea. In the late eighteenth and early nineteenth centuries, wealthy Europeans were enamored of everything oriental. People had to have more than just tea imported from the east—they had to have tea ware as well. Impressionist painters such as Monet, Cézanne, and Renoir were influenced by Japanese art prints (which had originally come to France as wrapping paper for imported goods), and by the tea ware that displayed images of nature such as birds and trees. The painters began to copy the Japanese style of allowing brush strokes to show, and of painting scenes *en plein air,* or outdoors (as opposed to portraits and landscapes done inside artists' studios).

Tea in England

✳ The first real evidence of tea in England was in the form of an ad in a newspaper by Thomas Garway in 1658. It read in part, "That excellent and by all physicians approved drink called by Chineans tcha, by other nations Tay alias Tea is sold at the Sultaness Head a Cophee house in Sweetings Rents by the Royal Exchange London." Some of his claims about the benefits of tea included:

◆ It maketh the Body active and lusty.

◆ It helpeth the Head-ach, giddiness and heaviness thereof.

◆ It removeth the Obstructions of the Spleen.

◆ It removeth Lassitude, and cleareth and purifieth adult Humors and hot Liver.

◆ It is good against Crudities, strengthening the weakness of the Ventricle or Stomack, causing good Appetite and Digestion, and particularly for Men of corpulent Body and such as are the great eaters of Flesh.

◆ It vanquisheth heavy Dreams, easeth the Brain, and strengtheneth the Memory.

◆ It overcometh superfluous Sleep, and prevents Sleepiness in general, a draught of the Unfusion being taken, so that without trouble whole nights may be spend in study without hurt to the Body, in that it moderately healeth and bindeth the mouth of the stomach.

◆ It is good for Colds, Dropsies and Scurveys, if properly infused purging the Blood of Sweat and Urine, and expelleth Infection.

✳ When Garway first began selling tea, it was very expensive: it sold for sixteen shillings per pound or about five continental dollars for the time. By the end of the 1700s, tea had become popularized, and the price dropped to one-fifth of a shilling per pound.

✳ Garway is also credited with the first acknowledgment in England of the use of milk in tea. He writes, "being prepared with milk and water strengthen the inward parts." Milk was not originally used in tea in England as it is today. Instead they added saffron, ginger, nutmeg, and salt. It has also been said, although it has never been documented, that the use of milk in tea might have come from the Mongols, who to this day mix hot milk with their tea. This practice was eventually brought into China and the practice was then taken abroad via the Dutch East India Trading Company, which is where the French probably adopted it.

* In 1702, Queen Anne announced that she preferred to drink tea rather than ale in the morning for breakfast. She is also credited with using silver teapots rather than Chinese ceramic pots. This was the first major change in the use of tea in England; it created a tremendous demand for tea, as well as an unprecedented demand for English silver tea service sets.

* Black tea replaced green tea coming from China. Black tea, which is oxidized, keeps much longer than green tea. This was an important consideration in the days when it could take many weeks or months for the tea to make it to Europe and England from China.

* In 1706, Thomas Twining began to serve tea at Tom's Coffee House in London. By 1717, it had evolved into the first teashop, called the Golden Lyon, which began a new custom—allowing both men and women to patronize the shop.

* The Opium Wars: Tea became so popular with the English by the mid 1700s, they were importing over 4.5 million tons of black tea a year. Paying for this tea was creating a burden on the currency reserves in England. The government saw its answer in the opium crops of India, a British-controlled colony. Early in the nineteenth century, British merchants began smuggling opium into China in order to balance their purchases of tea for export to Britain. In 1839, China destroyed a large quantity of opium confiscated from British merchants. Great Britain responded by sending gunboats to attack several Chinese coastal cities. China was defeated and forced to sign treaties that opened many of its ports to British trade. In 1856, a second war broke out. China was again defeated and was

compelled to accept more treaties, to which France, Russia, and the United States were also party, opening even more ports to trade.

✳ In 1840, Anna, the Duchess of Bradford, started the custom of afternoon tea in England. At the time, the English would have a small breakfast in the morning, and then not dine again until eight or nine o'clock at night. As a result, they were often hungry in the afternoon. The Duchess, noticing that every afternoon she would have a "sinking feeling," began to order a small meal of bread, butter, cakes, tarts, and biscuits, to be brought secretly to her boudoir. She thought that if discovered, she would be ridiculed—but it turned out everyone else was hungry, too, and her idea caught on with the masses. In an historical coincidence, the Duchess conceived the idea of afternoon tea at approximately the same time that the Earl of Sandwich came up with the idea of putting a filling between two slices of bread. . . .

TEASER

Hand-Me-Down Tea

In the 1700s and 1800s, tea was a luxury item kept in only the richest households. The wealthy prized their tea, and kept it locked away in tea chests. They would resteep the tea several times. After a few steeps, the servants would take the tea leaves and use them to make tea for themselves. After they steeped the tea, they would sell the used leaves to street vendors, who would press the leaves into tea cakes (sometimes mixed with manure from the horses in the street). They were sold to people who could only afford to spend a penny or two for tea.

It is from these street vendors that we get the phrase "tea for two." The vendors usually sold a pot of tea for three pence, or thruppence. But if they wanted to drum up business, they would sometimes lower the price to tuppence, or two pence, by yelling, "Tea for two."

Tea in India

* The *Camellia sinensis* plant is native to India; however, it was not identi-fied until the early 1800s. As a result of the Opium Wars, the British were looking for ways to decrease their dependence on China for tea, so in 1778, British naturalist Sir Joseph Banks, hired by the East India Company, suggested that India grow tea plants imported from China. Although they tried for fifty years, they were mostly unsuccessful, as they did not grow well in India's warmer climate.

* Between 1815 and 1831, East India Company botanists came to recog-nize that there were, in fact, indigenous Indian tea plants.

* In 1835, the East India Company organized its first tea plantation in Assam, India.

* The first auction of tea grown in India was held in London in 1838; however, the tea was from Chinese plants they had finally managed to grow in India.

* In 1856, Chinese tea was planted in and around Darjeeling, India, and grew very well. Darjeeling tea became one of the best and most prized teas of the Chinese varieties.

* In the late 1800s, after the Opium Wars, China would no longer provide England with any tea. The Indian tea market blossomed. To-day India produces more tea than any other country except for China.

Tea in America: How Tea Shaped Our Country

* In 1650, tea was introduced to the Dutch colony of New Amsterdam (later New York) by Peter Stuyvesant. It is said this colony enjoyed tea before it was ever introduced in England.

* The British took over New Amsterdam in 1664 and renamed it New York. They found that the colony was already drinking more green tea than they were in England.

* By 1765, tea was the most popular beverage in the American colonies.

* In 1767, British Parliament passed the Townsend Revenue Act, imposing a tax on the tea and other commodities imported into the British colonies. This had a lot to do with additional revenues needed to finance England's own consumption of tea from China.

* In 1770, the tax on all items—except tea—was repealed.

* Women saved the day! They united and decided not to purchase any tea. This action was taken to heart by women throughout the colonies so that tea would never be unloaded off boats in any port.

* On December 16, 1773, 5,000 colonists met to determine what should be done about the tea tax. That night, fifty men dressed as Indians attacked the three British ships in Boston Harbor and dumped over forty tons of green tea into the harbor. Similar acts erupted in Philadelphia, New York, Maine, North Carolina, and Maryland through 1774.

* The British made several attempts to put down the rebellion, but in 1776 the American Revolution began.

* George Washington was an avid tea drinker and was provided three cups of tea every morning, even during the war. He continued the practice of having three cups of green tea at breakfast during his tenure as president.

* In the 1830s, clipper ships were introduced to the high seas. The ships' bows were distinctively narrow and heavily raked forward, which allowed them to rapidly cut or clip through the waves. The creation of the clipper ships added speed to the arrival of teas from China. This was crucial to the freshness of the teas, which made for a better taste. Additionally, the

clipper ships brought Chinese labor to the United States, which helped build our country. The best known of these ships were the China clippers, also known as tea clippers, designed to sail the trade routes between Europe and the East Indies. The last surviving example of these ships was the *Cutty Sark,* which was preserved in drydock in Greenwich, England. Unfortunately, it suffered extensive damage in a fire on May 21, 2007.

✳ Tea gave rise to millionaires: Some of the first American millionaires made their fortunes from tea. John Jacob Astor, the first millionaire in the United States, T. H. Perkins, an enormously wealthy Boston merchant, and Stephen Girard of Philadelphia, known as the "gentle tea merchant," made fortunes trading tea with China. They sold the tea through retailers like the Great Atlantic and Pacific Tea Company—which became known as A&P, the country's first supermarket chain.

✳ The most famous story of how iced tea was invented goes like this: British plantation owner and tea merchant Richard Blechynden brought black tea to the 1904 St. Louis World's Fair, planning to give away free samples of hot tea. But it was so hot outside, no one was interested. So he came up with the idea of pouring the tea over ice . . . and the rest is history. However, there are recorded instances of people drinking iced tea before 1904. A newspaper article detailing the Missouri State Reunion of Ex-Confederate Veterans held in Nevada, Missouri on September 20 and 21, 1890, describes that the meal was "washed down with . . . 880 gallons of iced tea." And according to Pat Vilmer of the St. Louis World's Fair Society (as told to the World Green Tea Association), "The good people of the South were serving iced tea in their homes long before the Fair . . . It was called sweet tea served cool not hot in the summer in the South. Ice when available, was used. Remember, ice was the premium in the early days before refrigeration, not tea."

✳ The next American tea invention came from tea importer Thomas Sullivan. In order to provide samples of tea leaves for his customers, Sullivan packed them in hand-sewn silk pouches. The customers liked the convenience of these bags so much, they demanded to receive their tea in like style. So Sullivan replaced the silk with more economical gauze, and the tea bag was born.

TEASER

Want Faster Service?

Coffeehouses were popular gathering places in eighteenth century England, and became even more popular when they added tea to the menu. They were often called "Penny Universities" because for a penny you could get a pot of tea and a newspaper, and usually find someone with whom you could engage in an "important" conversation. Many traditions we still follow have their roots in these beverage shops. In one particular coffeehouse called the Turk's Head, many arguments arose. In order to settle these disputes, the owner would bring out an old wooden box and patrons would vote as to which side should win the argument. When democracy took hold, this became the template for the now familiar ballot box.

Often these coffeehouses would be so busy, patrons would find themselves with a long wait before being served. If they wanted to make sure they were served quickly, they would put money into a wooden box labeled T.I.P.: To Insure Promptness. Thus, the modern concept of tipping evolved.

TEAmmate Profile

Name: Meghan C.

Age: 23

Total Weight Loss: 12

Total Inches Lost: 16.5

Favorite Tea: Moroccan Mint

When I went to college, I took advantage of everything college had to offer—which included eating and drinking—and I just had gotten to a weight that was unhealthy. I already had a medical history, even at my age, so I wanted to lose weight just for my health. Plus, I wanted to look better.

I have a pretty busy work schedule. I'm a production assistant at a TV show. There's a lot of running around. During the day, I switched to taking the stairs even before I started the diet, and I work on the seventh floor. After starting the diet, I joined a gym. I was a runner before; I used to run track. I started off running four miles a day. Now I'm running anywhere from seven to eight miles a day.

Like a lot of places in this business, we always have food around. And a lot of unhealthy food. When it's right there at your fingertips, it's hard not to eat it. So I gained a lot of weight this season just working on my show. Bad food was in my face all the time. In the morning, I'd have cereal or a bagel, maybe some fruit, and always a couple of cups of coffee. Lunch would be ordered in from somewhere in the neighborhood, usually sandwiches. Dinner was very sporadic. I'd pick something up on the way home, or anything that was left over from the lunch at the office. Or I'd make a can of soup.

Since I went on the diet, I started having yogurt in the morning with some fruit, or egg whites with a piece of ham and a slice of nonfat cheese. When I did want some carbs, especially when I was running a lot, I'd have a whole-wheat English muffin or some oatmeal with some fresh fruit in it. Lunch was the hardest meal to switch. I stopped going for the free food and started bringing my own healthier food. Sometimes I'd just make a sandwich with a couple of slices of turkey and some veggies. Sometimes I would order out from work, I'd get a salad or a piece of salmon with some sauce on the side.

Dinner was also a really big change. My roommate and I—she's also on the diet—started cooking for ourselves. All fresh fruit, all fresh vegetables. Chicken, or meatballs. We used a lot of the recipes we got from Dr. Tea. At the beginning we were a little leery of cooking with tea. But we tried all the rubs and loved them. Any time we steam vegetables, we use tea. Any time you use water in a recipe, we use tea instead.

At the beginning, it was difficult to make all these changes. But then I would drink the tea and that would help me not eat all day. When I first started, it was really hard to give up coffee. I gave it up cold turkey after the first meeting and I haven't had a cup since. I replaced my two cups of coffee in the morning with two cups of tea. Then I usually have another cup of tea after I've had breakfast. It fills me up. I have one or two before lunch, depending on how busy my day is. Sometimes it was hard when I was running around doing errands for work. But then I just started carrying a large water bottle with me filled with tea. Then my roommate and I got these large jugs of water with a spigot. We drain it, use the water to make tea, refill it with the tea, and then we have it in the refrigerator with tea already in it. So instead of having to make tea for each small water bottle, we just open the spigot, fill up a water bottle right from the fridge and we're ready to go.

One of the reasons I like this diet is because it definitely requires you to have some "me" time. I have this very busy job where I cater to a lot of people. I wasn't really taking care of myself. I'd come home and I'd crash. I was just very tired all the time. I didn't feel good, physically or mentally. Because of the diet I started making time to work out and I started eating better. I became more conscious about decisions I was making. I stopped drinking beer, which, as a young person, was a bit hard to deal with—all that peer pressure. But I feel so much better now. I'm less tired. My body feels better. I feel like I can do more things.

13

Epilogue

I t's amazing how life goes around in circles. My family has been in the tea business for well over 200 years. My grandfather was one of the biggest distributors of teas in the Middle East. He was a wholesaler, and though he dealt with many other commodities, his passion was for tea. When he was a merchant in Iraq, there was no television, no movies. As it was in most of the Middle East, social life centered around tea. In the 1950s, my grandfather, sensing that it was time to leave, moved his sons out of the Middle East. And my family more or less left the tea behind.

My father, who eventually became an accountant, started drinking coffee because everyone in America drank coffee. My grandfather still drank tea, and so did my mother's parents, but it was no longer the center of social life. We had both tea and coffee in the house and drank them both equally.

I grew up neither interested nor uninterested in tea. It was a part of my history, but nothing more.

However, as I grew up, I discovered that I was a man of nose and palate— which means I love all things related to the senses. I have always loved food and the intricacies of cooking. I became a connoisseur of fine foods, wines, spirits, beers, and tobacco. I'm one of those people who gets passionate about things. I can't help it; it's who I am.

When I started to make changes in my life, when I gave up coffee and started drinking tea, it became not only my passion, but my life. Now, every time my father walks into dr. tea's, he laughs at how life has come full circle, from his father to his son.

Writing this book has been an incredible journey and an honor for me, and I hope reading it has been one for you, too. It makes no difference to me if you lost 10 or 100 pounds. What matters to me is you have begun the process to change your life one cup of tea at a time.

Now that you've come to the end of the book, you have not come to the end of your journey. This is just the beginning. You can keep going down this new road you've just started traveling. All you have to do is remember: If I say I can, I will; if I say I can't I won't.

I would love to hear your test-TEA-monials. Please send me your stories. E-mail me if you have any questions. Come visit me at dr. tea's. Stay in touch; I look forward to hearing from you.

You are the new voice of the Ultimate Tea Diet!

Dr. Tea

dr. tea's

8612 Melrose Avenue

West Hollywood, CA 90069

1-310-657-9300

1-888-UTD-TEAS

drtea@ultimateteadiet.com

www.ultimateteadiet.com

www.doctor-tea.com

www.shopdrtea.com

ACKNOWLEDGMENTS

Rusty Robertson, for her vision, guidance, coaching, and extraordinary abilities in making the Ultimate Tea Diet, Dr. Tea, and dr. tea's a reality. You are truly one of a kind and I am most appreciative of your tireless efforts.

Mary Ellen O'Neill, my publisher, who go it! I am forever grateful MEO!

Sharyn Kolberg, for her words and oh so much more.

Christine Bybee and Pam Ross, for their expertise, time, and devotion to the Ultimate Tea Diet.

Paul Olsewski, Angie Lee, Janina Wong, Teresa Brady, Laura Dozier, and the entire HarperCollins Team.

Ed Robertson, Sue Schwartz, Angee Jenkins, Karen Reifschneider, Karen Saunders, and Woody Frasier, for your inexhaustible efforts.

All members of my Ultimate Tea Diet study group, who devoted eight weeks of their lives (now for the rest of their lives), who said I CAN, and they DID lose weight and inches, but more importantly confirmed that tea does change one's life in every way and for every age. For this I am forever proud to know each and every one of you.

Gram, for her love and devotion and showing that everything in life is better when love is added. I know you would be proud!

Grampa, for his big cup of tea each day.

My dad and my entire Ukra family from Baghdad, who started our tea business 200 years ago. Your dad and my grandfather would be proud.

My mom Charlotte, who never gave up on me.

My sis Tara MacMahon, for her lifelong devotion, and my brother-in law Paul MacMahon, for his guidance and wisdom.

Jan and Michael Schwartz, for always being there.

All of our family and friends, who are a constant source of love, support and encouragement.

All of our devoted dr. tea's family and staff, past and present, who make what we do every day so much fun.

Our spiritual teachers and inner ashram, whose guidance and wisdom has led us to where we are today.

Dr. Robert Gerard, my teacher, who at 90 years old always believed in me, and whose teachings and guidance taught me the meditations and invocations that led us to dr. tea's, finding my true path in life, and planetary consciousness.

My two devoted loving assistants, Curly and Lulu, with whom I spent every hour researching and writing this book.

And Julie, my wife and partner for life, and Lucky, my daughter and constant teacher and my pride and joy, who provided me the encouragement to write this book. Their love and devotion and light allowed me the incentive to make this book a reality and for this I am forever grateful.

Resources

There are thousands of Web sites offering tea and tea accessories. Those listed below are just a few you might want to visit.

TEA

dr. tea's
www.ultimateteadiet.com
1-888-UTD-TEAS

CVS
www.cvs.com
1-888-607-4287

Dean & Deluca
www.deandeluca.com
1-800-221-7714

Lipton Tea
www.liptont.com
1-888-547.8668

Art of Tea
www.artoftea.com
1-877-268-8327

Tea Affair
www.tea-affair.com
1-866-832-7467

Red & Green Company
www.rngco.com
1-415-626-1375

Adagio Teas
www.adagio.com

Stash Tea
www.stashtea.com
1-503-603-9905

Republic of Tea
www.republicoftea.com
1-800-298-4832

Upton Tea
www.uptontea.com
1-800-234-8327

Tazo Tea
www.tazo.com
1-800-299-9445

Special Teas
www.specialteas.com
1-800-365-6983

Harney & Sons
www.harney.com
1-888-427-6398

The Tao of Tea
www.taooftea.com
1-503-736-0198

In Pursuit of Tea
www.inpursuitoftea.com
1-866-878-3832

Revolution Tea
www.revolutiontea.com
1-888-321-4738

Whole Foods Market
www.wholefoodsmarket.com
1-512-477-4455

Bigelow Teas
www.bigelowtea.com
1-888-244-3569

TEA ACCESSORIES

dr. tea's
www.ultimateteadiet.com
1-888-UTD-TEAS

Dean & Deluca
www.deandeluca.com
1-800-221-7714

Art of Tea
www.artoftea.com
1-877-268-8327

Bodum
www.bodum.com
1-800-232-6386

Stash Tea
www.stashtea.com
1-503-603-9905

Café de Fiori
www.cafedefiori.com
1-818-901-7777

The Tao of Tea
www.taooftea.com
1-503-736-0198

Bigelow Teas
www.bigelowtea.com
1-888-244-3569

SpecialTeas
www.specialteas.com
1-800-365-6983

These days, your local supermarket probably carries a wide variety of teas in a vast array of flavors. Here are just a few you may find in a store near you (and if you can't, try their Web sites):

Dr. Tea's Ultimate Tea Diet Teas
www.ultimateteadiet.com

Lipton Tea
www.liptont.com

Rishi Tea
www.rishi-tea.com

Two Leaves and a Bud
www.worldpantry.com

Republic of Tea
www.republicoftea.com

Triple Leaf Tea
www.tripleaf-tea.com

Mighty Leaf Tea
www.mightyleaf.com

Stash Tea
www.stash.com

Twinings Tea
www.twinings.com

Allegro Tea
www.allegrocoffee.com

Yogi Tea
www.yogitea.com

Golden Moon Tea
www.goldenmoontea.com

References

Adhami, V. M., N. Ahmad, and H. Mukhtar. Molecular targets for green tea in prostate cancer prevention. *Journal of Nutrition* 2003 July; 133 (7):2417S–2424S. Abstract available at http://www.nutrition.org/cgi/content/abstract/133/7/2417S.

Ahmad, N., et al. Antioxidants in chemoprevention of skin cancer. *Current Problems on Dermatology* 2001; 29:128–39.

Ahmad, N., et al. Green tea polyphenols and cancer: biologic mechanism and practical implications. *Nutrition Revision* 1999 March; 57(3):78–83.

Ahmed, S., et al. Green tea polyphenol epigallocatechin-3-gallate (EGCG) differentially inhibits interleukin-1β-induced expression of matrix metalloproteinase-1 and -13 in human chondrocytes. *Journal of Pharmacology And Experimental Therapeutics* 2004; 308(2):767–73.

Anderson, R.A., and M.M. Polansky. Tea enhances insulin activity. *Journal of Agricultural and Food Chemistry* 2002 Nov; 50(24):7182–6.

Arteel, G.E., T. Uesugi, et al. Green tea extract protects against early alcohol-induced liver injury in rats. *Biological Chemistry* 2002 Mar–Apr; 383(3–4): 663–70.

Aschan, Stefan. "Caffeine Exposed." *ABC News*, March 29, 2007. http://abcnews.go.com/Health/Diet/Story?id=2990014&page=1, accessed April 15, 2007.

Astrup, A., S. Toubro, et al. Caffeine: a double-blind, placebo-controlled study of its thermogenic, metabolic, and cardiovascular effects in healthy volunteers. *American Journal of Clinical Nutrition* 1990; 51:759–67.

Baker, J.A., et al. Consumption of black tea or coffee and risk of ovarian cancer. *International Journal of Gynecological Cancer* 2007 Jan/Feb; 17(1):50–54.

Banerjee, S., P. Maity, et al. Black tea prevents cigarette smoke-induced apoptosis and lung damage. *Journal of Inflammation* 2007 April; 4(1):3.

Bell, S.J., et al. A functional food product for the management of weight. *Critical Reviews in Food Science and Nutrition* 2002; 42(2):163–78.

Bettuzzi, S., M. Brausi, et al. Chemoprevention of human prostate cancer by oral administration of green tea catechins in volunteers with high-grade prostate intraepithelial neoplasia: a preliminary report from a one-year proof-of-principle study. *Cancer Research* 2006 Jan.; 66(2):1234–40.

"Black Tea Soothes Away Stress." *BBC News* October 4, 2006. http://news .bbc.co.uk/2/hi/health/5405686.htm.

Bliss, Rosalie Marion. Brewing up the latest tea research. *Agricultural Research*. Sept. 2003:11–13.

Bukowski, J.F. et al. Human gamma-delta T cells recognize alkylamines derived from microbes, edible plants, and tea: implications for innate immunity. *Immunity* 1999 July; 11(1):57–65.

"Caffeine Nation." *CBS News*. September 7, 2003. http://www.cbsnews.com/ stories/2002/11/14/sunday/main529388.shtml, accessed May 6, 2007.

"Caffeine: How Much is Too Much?" http://www.mayoclinic.com/health/ caffeine/NU00600 accessed April 1, 2007.

Cao, H., M. A. Kelly, et al. Green tea increases anti-inflammatory tristetraprolin and decreases pro-inflammatory tumor necrosis factor mRNA levels in rats. *Journal of Inflammation* 2007; 4:1. http://www.journal-inflammation.com/content/4/1/1.

Chantre, P., D. Lairon. Recent findings of green tea extract AR25 (exolise) and its activity for the treatment of obesity. *Phytomedicine* 2002 Jan; 9(1):3–8.

Cherniske, Stephen, *Caffeine Blues: Wake Up to the Hidden Dangers of America's #1 Drug*. New York: Warner Books, 1998.

Das, M. et al. Studies with black tea and its constituents on leukemic cells and cell lines. *Journal of Experimental & Clinical Cancer Research* 2002; 21(4):563–8.

Davies, M. J., J. T. Judd, et al. Black tea consumption reduces total and LDL cholesterol in mildly hypercholesterolemic adults. *Journal of Nutrition* 2003; 133:3298S–3302S.

Doheny, Kathleen. Pros and cons of the caffeine craze. http://www.webmd.com/content/Article/128/117161.htm, accessed May 2, 2007.

Duffy, S.J., et al. Short- and long-term black tea consumption reverses endothelial dysfunction in patients with coronary artery disease. *Circulation* 2001; 104:151–6.

Dulloo A.G., C. Duret, et al. Efficacy of a green tea extract rich in catechin polyphenols and caffeine in increasing 24-h energy expenditure and fat oxidation in humans. *American Journal of Clinical Nutrition* 1999 Dec; 70:1040–45.

Dulloo A.G., J. Seydoux, et al. Green tea and thermogenesis: interactions between catechin-polyphenols, caffeine, and sympathetic activity. *International Journal of Obesity and Related Metabolic Disorders* 2000 Feb; 24(2):252–8.

Dulloo, A.G., C.A. Geissler, et al. Normal caffeine consumption: influence on thermogenesis and daily energy expenditure in lean and postobese human volunteers. *American Journal of Clinical Nutrition* 1989; 49(1):44–50.

Egashira, N., K. Hayakawa, et al. Neuroprotective effect of gamma-glutamylethylamide (theanine) on cerebral infarction in mice. *Neuroscience Letters* 2004 June 3; 363(1):58–61.

Ganio, M.S., et al. Evidence-based approach to lingering hydration questions. *Clinics in Sports Medicine* 2007 Jan; 26(1):1–16.

Geleijnse, J.M., et al. Inverse association of tea and flavonoid intakes with incident myocardial infarction: the Rotterdam study. *American Journal of Clinical Nutrition* 2002; 75(5):880–6.

Genesee Country Health Department Staff. Beware of caffeine in energy drinks. *Flint Journal* April 30, 2007; http://www.mlive.com/entertainment/fljournal/index.ssf?/base/features-6/1177941143183520.xml&coll=5, accessed May 2, 2007.

Gilbert, Monica. Tea Leaves Promise Well-Being. *The Natural Foods Merchandiser* Nov. 1, 2004; XXV(11):46–48.

Graham, H.N. Green tea composition, consumption, and polyphenols chemistry. *Preventive Medicine* 1992 May; 21(3):334–50.

Granato, Heather. It's Tea Time. *Natural Products Insider* May 26, 2003; http://www.naturalproductsinsider.com/articles/468/468_361fbff1 .html, accessed April 27, 2007.

"Green Tea and EGCG May Help Prevent Autoimmune Diseases." *Science Daily* April 20, 2007; http://www.sciencedaily.com/releases/2007/04/ 070419140910.htm.

University of Chicago Medical Center. Green tea derivative causes loss of appetite, weight loss in rats. Feb. 23, 2000; http://www.uchospitals.edu/ news/2000/20000223-tea.html.

"Green tea may keep HIV at bay." *BBC News* March 29, 2007; http://news .bbc.co.uk/go/pr/fr/-/2/hi/health/6502399.stm, accessed April 6, 2007.

Greider, Katherine, and Roberta Yared. Debunking Decaf. *AARP Bulletin* December 2006.

Gupta S., T. Hussain, et al. Molecular pathway for (-)-epigallocatechin-3-gallate-induced cell cycle arrest and apoptosis of human prostate carcinoma cells. *Archives of Biochemistry and Biophysics* 2003 Feb 1; 410(1):177–85.

Gupta, S., B. Saha, et al. Comparative antimutagenic and anticlastogenic effects of green tea and black tea: a review. *Mutation Research* 2002; 512(1)37–65.

Hakim, I., R. Harris, et al. Effect of increased tea consumption on oxidative DNA damage among smokers: a randomized controlled study. *Journal of Nutrition* 2003 Oct; 133(10):3303S–3309S.

Han, L.J., T. Takaku, et al. Anti-obesity action of oolong tea. *International Journal of Obesity* 1999 Jan; 23(1):98–105.

Haqqi, T.M., et al. Prevention of collagen-induced arthritis in mice by a polyphenolic fraction from green tea. *Proceedings of the National Academy of Sciences* 1999 April 13; 96(8):4524–29.

Hegarty, V.M., et al. Tea drinking and bone mineral density in older women. *American Journal of Clinical Nutrition* 2000; 71:1003–7.

Hindmarch, I., P.T. Quinlan, et al. The effects of black tea and other beverages on aspects of cognition and psychomotor performance. *Psychopharmacology* 1998; 139(3):230–8.

Hirano, R., Y. Momiyama, et al. Comparison of green tea intake in Japanese patients with and without angiographic coronary artery disease. *American Journal of Cardiology* 2002 Nov. 15; 90:1150–53.

Hodgson, J.M. Effects of tea and tea flavonoids on endothelial function and blood pressure: a brief review. *Clinical and Experimental Pharmacology and Physiology* 2006 Sept; 33(9):838–41.

Hollman, P.C.H., et al. The addition of milk to tea does not affect the absorption of flavonoids from tea in man. *Free Radical Research* 2001 March; 34(3):297–300.

Hsu, S., W. Bollag, et al. Green tea polyphenols induce differentiation and proliferation in epidermal keratinocytes. *Journal of Pharmacology And Experimental Therapeutics* 2003; 306:29–34.

Hsu, S., D. Dickinson, et al. Inhibition of autoantigen expression by (-)-epigallocatechin-3-gallate (the major constituent of green tea) in normal human cells. *Journal of Pharmacology And Experimental Therapeutics* 2005 July 26; 315:805–811.

Hurley Deriso, Christine. Green tea linked to skin cell rejuvenation. Medical College of Georgia, February 3, 2006; http://www.mcg.edu/news/2003news-rel/hsu.htm, accessed April 25, 2007.

Ikeda, I., R. Hamamoto, et al. Dietary gallate esters of tea catechins reduce deposition of visceral fat, hepatic triaglycerol, and activities of hepatic enzymes related to fatty acid synthesis in rats. *Bioscience, Biotechnology, and Biochemistry* 2005; 69(5):1049–53.

Imai, K., K. Suga, et al. Cancer-preventative effects of drinking tea among a Japanese population. *Preventive Medicine* 1997 Nov–Dec; 26(6):769–75.

Isaacson, Andy. Steeped in Tea: The Social Significance of One Hot Drink. *Utne Reader,* Jan–Feb 2007; 51–57.

Juhel, C., M. Armand, et al. Green tea extract (AR25) inhibits lipolysis of triglycerides in gastric and duodenal medium in vitro. *Journal of Nutritional Biochemistry* 2000 Jan; 11(1):45–51.

Kakuda, T, et al. Inhibiting effects of theanine on caffeine stimulation evaluated by EEG in the rat. *Bioscience, Biotechnology, and Biochemistry* 2000 Feb; 64:287–93.

Kakuda, T. Neuroprotective effects of the green tea components theanine and catechins. *Biological and Pharmaceutical Bulletin* 2002 Dec; 25(12): 1513–18.

Kallen, Ben. Fat loss in a tiny bag: if you belly runneth over, fill your cup with green tea to shrink it. *Men's Fitness.* Sept. 2002; http://www.findarticles .com/p/articles/mi_m1608/is_9_18/ai_9068387, accessed April 13, 2007.

Kamath, A.B., et al. Antigens in tea-beverage prine human Vγ2Vδ2 T cells in vitro and in vivo for memory and nonmemory antibacterial cytokine responses. *Proceedings of the National Academy of Science of the United States of America* 2003 May; 100(10):6009–14.

Katiyar, S.K. Skin photoprotection by green tea: antioxidant and immuno-modulatory effects. *Current Drug Targets. Immune Endocrine and Metabolic Disorders* 2003 Sep; 3(3):234–42.

Kiefer, Dale. Theanine: an amino acid from tea has numerous health-protecting effects. *Life Extension*, August 2005; http://lef.org/magazine/mag2005/ aug2005_aas_01.htm, accessed April 18, 2007.

Lane, J.D., et al. Caffeine impairs glucose metabolism in type 2 diabetes. *Diabetes Care* 2004 Aug; 27:2047–48. http://care.diabetesjournals.org/cgi/ content/extract/27/8/2047.

Lane, J.D., C.F. Pieper, et al. Caffeine affects cardiovascular and neuroendocrine activation at work and home. *Psychosomatic Medicine* 2002; 64(4): 595–603.

Larsson, S. C., A. Wolk. Tea consumption and ovarian cancer risk in a population-based cohort. *Archives of Internal Medicine* 2005 Dec; 165(22): 2683–86.

Leenan, R., et al. A single dose of tea with or without milk increase plasma antioxidant activity in humans. *European Journal of Clinical Nutrition* 2005 Jan; 54(1):87–92.

Leung, L.K., et al. Theaflavins in black tea and catechins in green tea are equally effective antioxidants. *Journal of Nutrition* 2001; 131(9):2248–51.

Liao, S. The medicinal action of androgens and green tea epigallocatechin gallate. *Hong Kong Medical Journal* 2001 Dec; 7(4):369–74.

Lindahl, B., I. Johansson, et al. Coffee drinking and blood cholesterol—effects of brewing method, food intake and life style. *Journal of Internal Medicine* 1991 Oct; 230(4):299–305.

"Look Younger Without Going Under the Knife." *Today, Weekend Edition* May 26, 2006; http://www.msnbc.msn.com/id/12645683, accessed October 26, 2006.

Lorenz, M., et al. Addition of milk prevents vascular protective effects of tea. *European Heart Journal* 2007 Jan; 28(2):219–23.

Lu, K., M.A. Gray, et al. The acute effects of L-theanine in comparison with alprazolam on anticipatory anxiety in humans. *Human Psychopharmacology* 2004 Oct; 19(7):457–65.

Lu, Y.P., Y.R. Lou, et al. Inhibitory effects of orally administered green tea, black tea, and caffeine on skin carcinogenesis in mice previously treated with ultraviolet B light (high risk mice): relationship to decreased tissue fat. *Cancer Research* 2001 July 1; 61(13):5002–9.

Maron, D.J., G. P. Lu, et al. Cholesterol-lowering effect of a theaflavin enriched green tea extract: a randomized controlled trial. *Archives of Internal Medicine* 2003 June 23; 163(12):1448–53.

Mason, R. 200 mg of Zen: L-theanine boosts alpha waves, promotes alert relaxation. *Alternative & Complementary Therapies* 2001 April; 7(2):91–95.

McCusker, R., B. Fuehrlein, et al. Technical note: caffeine content of decaffeinated coffee. *Journal of Analytical Toxicology* 2006 Oct; 30(8):611–13.

Murase, T., and S. Haramizu. Reduction of diet-induced obesity by a combination of tea-catechin intake and regular swimming. *International Journal of Obesity* (Lond) 2006 Mar; 30(3):561–8.

Murase, T. S. Haramizu, et al. Green tea extract improves endurance capacity and increases muscle lipid oxidation in mice. *American Journal of Physiology-Regulatory, Integrative and Comparative Physiology* 2005 Mar; 228(3): R708–15.

Murase, T., S. Haramizu, et al. Green tea extract improves running endurance in mice by stimulating lipid utilization during exercise. *American Journal of*

Physiology-Regulatory, Integrative and Comparative Physiology 2006 Jan; 290(6):R1550–56.

Nagao, T., et al. Ingestion of a tea rich in catechins leads to a reduction in body fat and malondialdehyde-modified LDL in men. *American Journal of Clinical Nutrition* 2005 Jan; 81(1):122–129.

Nakachi K., H. Eguchi, et al. Can teatime increase one's lifetime? *Ageing Research Reviews* 2003 Jan; 2(1):1–10.

Noriyasu, O., S. Satoko, et al. Effects of combination of regular exercise and tea catechins on energy expenditure in humans. *Journal of Health Science* 2005; 51(2):233–36.

Okakura, Kakuzo. *Book of Tea*. Mineola, NY: Dover Publications, 1964.

Okello, E.J., et al. In vitro anti-beta-secretase and dual anti-cholinesterase activities of Camellia sinensis L. (tea) relevant to treatment of dementia. *Phytotherapy Research* 2004 Aug; 18(8):624–27.

Ostrowska, J., W. Luczaj, et al. Green tea protects against ethanol-induced lipid peroxidation in rat organs. *Alcohol* 2004 Jan; 32(1):25–32.

Pajonk, F., A. Riedisser, et al. The effects of tea extracts on proinflammatory signaling. BMC Medicine 2006 Dec; 4:28.

Patenaude, Frédéric. Coffee: the great energy sapper. http://www.healthfree .com/raw_food_art_coffee.htm, accessed May 11, 2007.

Petrie, H.J., et al. 2004. Caffeine ingestion increases the insulin response to an oral-glucose-tolerance test in obese men before and after weight loss. *American Journal of Clinical Nutrition* July 2004; 80(1):22–28. http:// www.ajcn.org/cgi/content/abstract/80/1/22.

Perricone, Nicholas, MD. *The Perricone Prescription*. New York: HarperResource, 2002.

Quinan, P.T., Lane, J., et al. The acute physiological and mood effects of tea and coffee: the role of caffeine level. *Pharmacology Biochemistry and Behavior* 2000 May; 66(1):19–28.

Raloff, Janet. Trimming with tea. *Science News Online* February 12, 2005; 167(7). http://www.sciencenews.org/articles/20050212/food.asp, accessed April 14, 2007.

Rees, Judy R., Therese A. Stukel, et al. Tea consumption and basal cell and squamous cell skin cancer: results of a case-control study. *Journal of the American Academy of Dermatology* 2007 May; 56(5):781–85.

Roca, D.J., G.D. Schiller, and D.H. Farb. Chronic caffeine or theophylline exposure reduces gamma-aminubutyric acid/benzodiazepine receptor site interactions. *Molecular Pharmacology*, 1988 May; 33(5):481–85.

Rosick, Edward R. EGCG Can Help You Lose Weight. *Life Enhancement* December 1, 2005. http://www.life-enhancement.com/article_template. asp?id-1154, accessed October 10, 2006.

Rumpler, W., et al. Oolong tea increases metabolic rate and fat oxidation in men. *Journal Nutrition* 2001 Nov; 131(11):2848–52.

Salvaggio, A. M., Periti, et al. Coffee and cholesterol, an Italian study. *American Journal of Epidemiology* 1991; 134(2):149–56.

Sartippour M.R., D. Heber, et al. Green tea and its catechins inhibit breast cancer xenografts. *Nutrition and Cancer* 2001; 40(2):149–56.

Sartippour, M.R., Z. M. Shao, et al. Green tea inhibits vascular endothelial growth factor (VEGF) induction in human breast cancer cells. *Journal of Nutrition* 2002 Aug; 132(8):2307–11.

Sato D., and M. Matsushima. Preventive effects of urinary bladder tumors induced by N-butyl-N-(4-hydroxybutyl)-nitrosamine in rats by green tea leaves. *International Journal of Urology* 2003 March; 10(3):160–66.

Sato, Y., H. Nakatsuka, et al. Possible contribution of green tea drinking habits to the prevention of stroke. *Tohoku Journal of Experimental Medicine* 1989 Apr; 157(4):337–43.

Scott, Elizabeth, "Caffeine, Stress and Your Health: Is Caffeine Your Friend or Your Foe?" http://stress.about.com/od/stresshealth/a/caffeine.htm?p=1, accessed May 1, 2007.

Sesso, H.D., J.M. Gaziano, et al. Coffee and tea intake and the risk of myocardial infarction. *American Journal of Epidemiology* 1999 Jan; 149(2):162–67.

Setiawan, V.W., A. Zhang, et al. Protective effect of free tea on the risks of chronic gastritis and stomach cancer. *International Journal of Cancer* 2001; 92(4):600–604.

Shimotoyodome, A., S. Haramizu, et al. Exercise and green tea extract stimulate fat oxidation and prevent obesity in mice. *Medicine and Science in Sports Exercise* 2005 Nov; 37(11):1884–92.

Skrzydlewska, E., J. Ostrowska, et al. Green tea as a potent antioxidant in alcohol intoxication. *Addiction Biology* 2002 July; 7(3):307–314.

Song, C.H., et al. Effects of theanine on the release of brain alpha waves in adult males. *Korean Journal of Nutrition* 2003; 36(9):918–23.

Steptoe, A., E.L. Gibson, et al. The effects of tea on psychophysiological stress responsivity and post-stress recovery: a randomized double-blind trial. *Psychopharmacology* 2007 Jan; 190(1):81–89.

"Study: Drinking Coffee Has Health Benefits." August 28, 2005. http://abcnews.go.com/GMA/health/story?id=1074559, accessed Oct,1, 2006.

Sugiyama T. and Y. Sadzuka. Theanine and glutamate transporter inhibitors enhance the antitumor efficacy of chemotherapeutic agents. *Biochimica at Biophysica Actai Reviews on Cancer* 2003 Dec; 1653(2):47–59.

Taillefer, Theresa. Does coffee or caffeine affect my diabetes? Ask the Dietitian (Diabetes Dialogue, Winter 1997) http://www.diabetes.ca/Section_About/caffeine.asp, accessed April 15, 2007.

"Tea 'healthier' drink than water." *BBC News* August 24, 2006. http://news.bbc.co.uk/2/hi/health/5281046.stm, accessed April 4, 2007.

"Tea Snobs and Coffee Bigots." *New York Times* November 30, 1983. http://select.nytimes.com/search/restricted/article?res=F50A13F63A5D0C738FDDA80994DB484D81, accessed May 25, 2007.

Tsubono, Y., Y. Nishino, et al. Green tea and the risk of gastric cancer in Japan. *New England Journal of Medicine* 2001 Mar 1; 344(9):632–36.

Tuomilehto, J., G. Hu, et al. Coffee consumption and risk of type 2 diabetes mellitus among middle-aged finnish men and women. *JAMA* 2004 March; 291(10):1213–19.

Van het Hof, K.H., et al. Bioavailability of catechins from tea: the effect of milk. *Eur Journal Clinical Nutrition* 1998 May; 52(5):356–59.

Vayalil P.K., A. Mittal, et al. Green tea polyphenols prevent ultraviolet light-induced oxidative damage and matrix metalloproteinases expression in mouse skin. *Journal of Investigative Dermatology* 2004 Jun; 122(6):1480–7.

Vergote, D., C. Cren-Olivé, et al. (-)-Epigallocatechin (EGC) of green tea induces apoptosis of human breast cancer cells but not of their normal counterparts. *Breast Cancer Research and Treatment* 2002 Dec; 76(3):195–201.

Vijayakum, C., G.V. Reddy, et al. Addition of milk does not alter the antioxidant activity of black tea. *Annals of Nutrition and Metabolism* 2005 May–Jun; 49(3):189–95.

Wang, Y.C., and U. Bachrach. The specific anti-cancer activity of green tea (-)-epigallocatechin-3-gallate (EGCG). *Amino Acids* 2002 March; 22(2):131–43.

Wansink, Brian. *Mindless Eating: Why We Eat More Than We Think*. New York: Bantam, 2006.

Weil, Andrew, and Winifred Rosen. *From Chocolate to Morphine: Everything You Need to Know About Mind-Altering Drugs*. Boston: Houghton Mifflin, 2004.

Weisburger, J.H., E. Veliath, et al. Tea polyphenols inhibit the formation of mutagens during the cooking of meat. *Mutation Research* 2002 Apr 26; 516(1-2):19–22.

Westerterp-Plantenga, M.S., et al. Body weight loss and weight maintenance in relation to habitual caffeine intake and green tea supplementation. *Obesity Research* 2005; 13(7):1195–1204.

Wolfram, S., Y. Wang, et al. Anti-obesity effects of green tea: from bedside to bench. *Molecular Nutrition & Food Research* 2006 Feb; 50(2):176–87.

Yokozawa T., and E. Dong. Influence of green tea and its three major components upon low-density lipoprotein oxidation. *Experimental and Toxicologic Pathology* 1997 Dec; 49(5):329–35.

Yokozawa, T., T. Nakagawa, et al. Antioxidative activity of green tea polyphenols in cholesterol-fed rats. *Journal of Agricultural and Food Chemistry* 2002; 50(12):3549–52.

Zhang, M., et al., Green tea and the prevention of breast cancer: a case-control study in southeast China. *Carcinogenesis* 2007 28(5): 1074–78. Advance access December 20, 2006 at http://carcin.oxfordjournals.org.

Zhang M., C.W. Binns, et al. Tea consumption and ovarian cancer risk: a case-control study in China. *Cancer Epidemiology Biomarkers & Prevention* 2002 Aug; 11(8):713–18.

Zheng G., K. Sayama, et al. Anti-obesity effects of three major components of green tea, catechins, caffeine and theanine, in mice. *In Vivo* 2004 Jan–Feb; 18(1):55–62.

Zhou, J.R., et al. Soy phytochemicals and tea bioactive components synergistically inhibit androgen-sensitive human prostate tumors in mice. *Journal of Nutrition* 2003 Feb; 133(2):516–21.

SUBJECT INDEX

RECIPE INDEX